# PERUVIAN
# POWER FOODS

# ⊰ PERUVIAN ⊱
# POWER FOODS

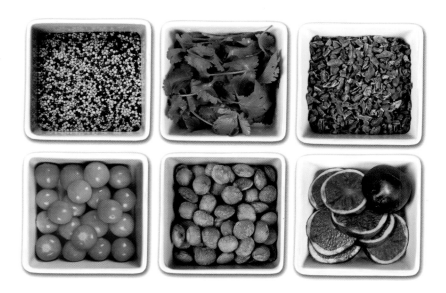

## 18 Superfoods, 101 Recipes, and
## Anti-aging Secrets from the Amazon to the Andes

Author of *Eating Free*
## Manuel Villacorta, MS, RD
and Jamie Shaw

**Health Communications, Inc.**
**Deerfield Beach, Florida**

*www.hcibooks.com*

DISCLAIMER: The information contained in this book is not intended as a substitute for the advice and/or medical care of the reader's physician, nor is it meant to discourage or dissuade the reader from the advice of his or her physician. The reader should consult with a physician in matters relating to his or her health and especially with regard to symptoms that may require a diagnosis. Any eating or lifestyle regimen should not be undertaken without first consulting with the reader's physician.

**Library of Congress Cataloging-in-Publication Data**

Villacorta, Manuel.
   Peruvian power foods : 18 superfoods, 101 recipes, and anti-aging secrets from the Amazon to the Andes / Manuel Villacorta and Jamie Shaw.
       p. cm.
   Includes bibliographical references and index.
   ISBN-13: 978-0-7573-1722-4 (Paperback)
   ISBN-10: 0-7573-1722-7 (Paperback)
   ISBN-13: 978-0-7573-1723-1(ePub)
   ISBN-10: 0-7573-1723-5 (ePub)
   1. Cooking, Peruvian.   2. Natural foods.   3. Nutrition.   4. Aging—Prevention.
I. Shaw, Jamie, MFA.   II. Title.
TX716.P4V56 2013
641.59'8544—dc23

                                         2013025633

Publisher:  Health Communications, Inc.
             3201 S.W. 15th Street
             Deerfield Beach, FL 33442-8190

*Cover design by Larissa Hise Henoch*
*Interior book design by Larissa Hise Henoch*
*Inside book formatting by Lawna Oldfield and Larissa Hise Henoch*
*Photography by Manuel Villacorta*

FOR THOSE READY TO OPTIMIZE
THEIR HEALTH USING SOME OF THE MOST
POWERFUL FOODS ON THE PLANET, THIS
BOOK IS DEDICATED TO YOU.

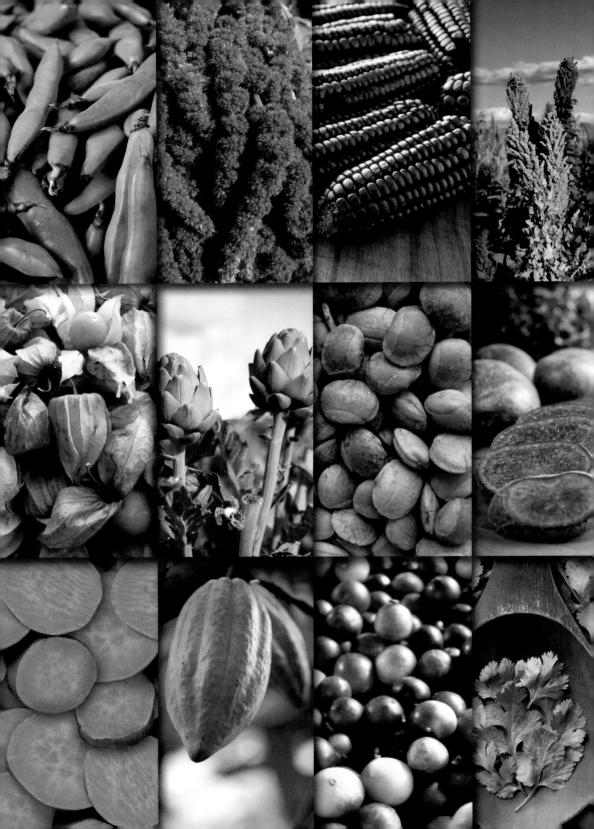

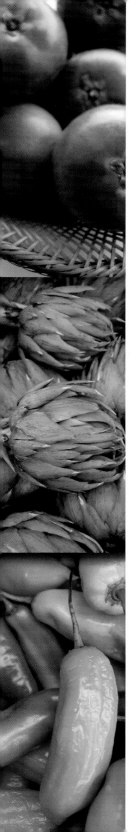

# A Culinary Word from
## ⁓ GASTÓN ACURIO ⁓

**FOR THOUSANDS OF YEARS,** Peruvians have cultivated count-less foods that are the basis of the global food chain: tubers, grains, corn, peppers, tomatoes, peanuts, and more. But there were many hidden treasures that remained undiscov-ered. Besides offering delicious, exotic flavors, these powerful ingredients provide incredible nutritional and medicinal benefits.

Today, Manuel Villacorta and Jamie Shaw reveal the secrets of these magical foods, adding to the great repertoire of Peruvian foods that has always been shared with the world. I am delighted to recommend this book because readers will learn about these foods, their considerable health benefits, and also the practical and delicious ways to incorporate these foods into everyday cooking.

**—Gastón Acurio, ambassador of Peruvian cuisine
chef and owner, Astrid y Gastón, Panchita, and La Mar**

Gastón Acurio is a world renowned chef and ambassador of Peruvian cuisine. He is the owner of many revered restaurants around the world, including Astrid y Gastón, Panchita, and La Mar. In 2013, his restaurant Astrid y Gastón was named on the San Pellegrino list of The World's 50 Best Restaurants. Acurio is credited with starting the gastronomical revolution in Peru.

# CONTENTS

# ☙ ACKNOWLEDGMENTS ☙

**THE AUTHORS WISH TO THANK** the following people, without whom we couldn't have completed this project: Allison Janse, our editor at HCI Books, for believing in the project and supporting our vision from the beginning; Kim Weiss, for helping with PR and media strategy; Larissa Henoch, for working so closely with us on layout and design; and literary agent Andrea Hurst, for shepherding the project.

We would also like to thank Manuel's office team, whose dedication and support allowed us to focus on the project: Kelly Powers, who assisted in the kitchen, with photography and recipe inspiration and tasting. We are grateful for Suzie Parada's tireless energy and efforts in researching ingredients and health benefits, and Irene Fung for her outstanding recipe nutrient analysis. Without your work, we couldn't have done ours. We are also indebted to Manuel's partner, Sarah Koszyk, at MV Nutrition, who held down the office and took care of clients while we were traveling and writing the book.

We are eternally grateful to a few culinary collaborators who shared some favorite dishes and inspired us in our own recipe creation. Thank you to Morena Cuadra and Morena Escardó, founders and authors of the PeruDelights blog and authors of the *Everything Pervuian* cookbook. Thank you to Jason D'Angelo, chef at Waterbar in San Francisco, for sharing your beautiful seafood creations. And we'd also like to thank Manuel's cousin, Natahli Giha, a Peruvian pastry chef for creating some choice confections. Lastly, we would like to thank Coco Torres Del Aguila, Manuel's childhood friend, who provided us with the best restaurant recommendations for Lima and Cuzco, which provided great inspiration.

We are eternally grateful to Manuel's mother, Elvira, who hosted and chauffered us in Lima, as well as dear family friend, Norma Zevallos, who fed us and taught us how to make traditional Amazonian dishes. Also, a nod to Hans, who graciously gave up his room. Finally, our thanks to Papito y Miguel for their unwavering support and eager willingness to taste our creations.

# ⌒ INTRODUCTION ⌒

**THIS BOOK IS A LABOR OF LOVE.** Love of health, food, country, and travel. When we first began working together, building Manuel's brand for his weight-loss program, Eating Free, we could not have imagined that five years later, we'd be traveling to Peru and scouring remote mountain and jungle locales

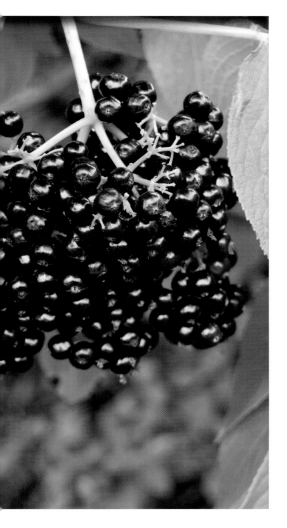

to learn more about the most powerful foods on the planet. But for Manuel—a registered dietitian and native Peruvian—and me, a writer drawn to food and travel—it was a dream project as well as a timely one.

For much of Manuel's career, he's focused on helping people embrace food, while teaching them how to lose weight safely and sensibly. Sadly, the American obesity epidemic keeps growing, and with it we see growing rates of diabetes, cancer, and heart disease. While health-conscious people used to focus primarily on how much to eat solely for weight maintenance, today we see an equally prevalent concern about which ingredients to eat for optimum health and disease-fighting potential. It's no longer enough to control calories or shrink portions when thinking about being totally healthy. To combat the effects of a toxic world, we must consider the quality and purity of what we're eating as well. This mind-set is bringing with it a paradigm shift away from quick and convenient foods and back toward the farmers' markets, organic food, and, of course, power foods.

We define power foods as hardworking functional foods that far surpass basic nutritional content. They are, quite simply, the cleanest, most powerful, antioxidant-rich, anti-aging foods available anywhere. While these ingredients have been staple foods for centuries in South America—particularly Peru—

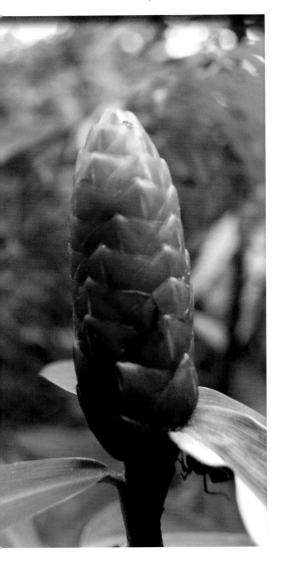

many of these foods are only newly available in the United States and elsewhere. Our goal is to introduce some of the most readily available choices, to reveal their nutritional and health benefits, and to share recipes that make it easy and enjoyable to integrate these amazing foods into your everyday diet.

You may have read in recent decades about the lower disease rates and longer life spans in some Asian and Mediterranean countries due to the high intake of produce, oils, and fish. We now know that adding ingredients classified as power foods to your diet can also offer incredible anti-aging health benefits. Please note, we don't use "anti-aging" to mean a wrinkle solution or some superficial promise. Rather, we're talking about a whole array of disease-fighting, immunity-strengthening ingredients that contribute to overall vitality and a long life.

Because these foods have long been hidden deep in Amazonian jungles and Andinian valleys, we are only beginning to understand their profound health

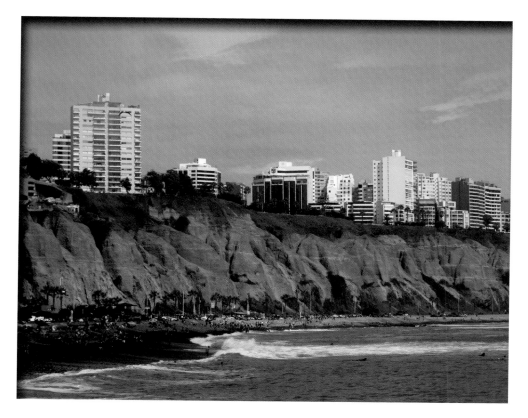

benefits. What we can unequivocally say is that they are proving to surpass even the wildest expectations of their potential healing properties. Many of the foods you'll learn about in this book have superlative health benefits, beating all other foods in their class with remarkable nutrient density. For example, the pichuberry is emerging as one of the most concentrated antioxidant fruits known to man. It has a remarkably low glycemic index (GI) of 25 (compared to a GI of 50 for blueberries and 53 for the pomegranate), so it's both a diabetic- and weight-loss-friendly fruit. Another superstar power food is sacha inchi oil, which packs the highest level of omega-3 fatty acids in any plant. By volume, sacha inchi has over 48 percent omega-3s—that's over 84 percent total fatty acids—so it's one of the most powerful inflammation fighters ever discovered. A third power food we'll introduce is camu camu, which is bursting with vitamin C (just one teaspoon can provide 1,180 percent of your daily vitamin C needs!). So as you can see, power foods aren't just a feel-good phenomenon. They are

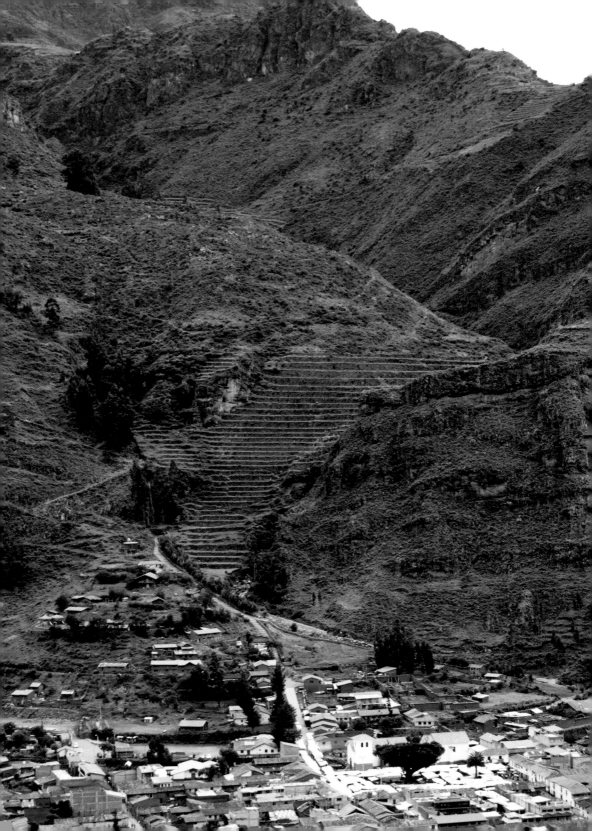

actually proving to be the most potent sources of dietary nutrition available to us. And while many people are already aware of this class of foods—perhaps from seeing them pop up in grocery stores or juice bars—most are still unsure about exactly what they are, what they do, and how to use them. That's why we set out on an adventure to discover the origins of and best uses for these incredibly potent foods.

We mapped a travel itinerary that would take us from the culinary capital of Lima, with its fresh seafood and *criollo* or traditional creations, to the rich farmlands of the Andes where over 3,000 kinds of potatoes and 200 species of corn are grown, to the depths of the Amazonian jungle, where thousands of potent fruits, nuts,

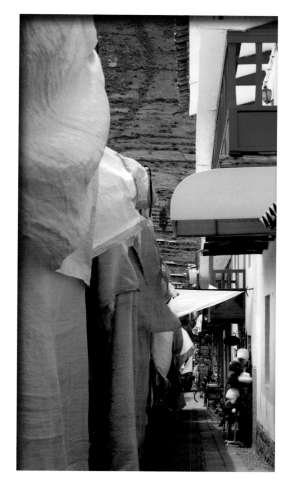

and seeds originate. Of course, Manuel came armed with all the latest scientific research about the properties of these ingredients, but we were also after the stories of these foods—where they come from, how they're prepared, and how the locals practice a farm-to-table approach. Our travels led us to open markets, restaurants, farms, home kitchens, and thatched jungle huts where we spoke to chefs, fishermen, farmers, *abuelitas*, aunties, food bloggers, and pretty much anyone else along the way who had a tale, some history, a recipe, or a recommendation about these foods. While we toured open markets in each area we visited, our experience culminated at the Belen Market in Iquitos, a bustling town on the river in the Amazonian jungle. Like the great markets of

India, the souks of Morocco, and the now-demolished stalls of Les Halles, the Belen Market is a city unto itself. Thousands of stalls deep, the marketplace is a destination for anything and everything, from exotic fruits and seeds to still-flapping piranhas and freshly poached monkey meat; from rattlesnakes and medicinal herbs from the local witchdoctor, to clothes and pills and fly-swatters. Belen is a microcosm of the greater city, with whole families sitting together selling wares, babies sleeping next to butchers plucking chickens, and rats scurrying under tables stacked high with pastries and plastic toys. Belen is, at once, third-world poverty and an explosion of Amazonian abun-

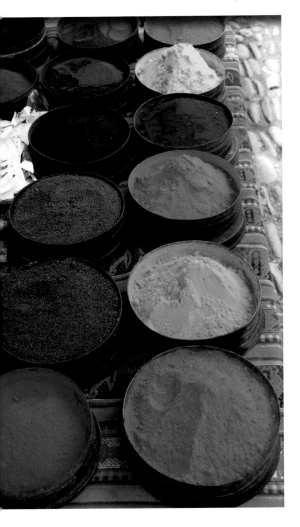

dance. The sheer amount of natural resources is staggering, and in some ways, it represents the rich offering of Peru at large. Here, we discovered foods we'd never seen, heard of, or tasted before—an indication of the still unknown resources and riches of this bountiful nation.

Part of the reason Peru is such a culinary hot spot is because its cuisine is an incredible fusion of local abundance and global flavor, from Mediterranean to Asian influences. Peru also boasts three distinct micro-climates. The rich topography spans the pristine coast, the fertile moun-tains and lush valleys, as well as the dense jungle rainforest.

Our goal in covering all this ground was to familiarize you with some of these exciting new foods (all of which are newly available in the United States) and encourage you to add as many of them as you're able to

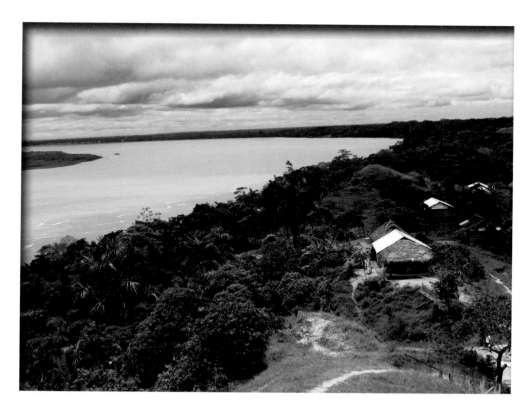

your regular diet. You'll gain the greatest benefit by mixing and matching these foods and eating them with regularity. In fact, be on the lookout for our "power-star" recipes—dishes that incorporate two or more power foods for the greatest health benefits in any one dish. It is, after all, the combination of all these nutrients and foods—not any one ingredient—that will offer you the optimal health benefit. Have fun and experiment, using these recipes as inspirational starting points. The dishes we've included range from the very simplest grab-and-go energy items, like smoothies, power bars, and raw truffles, to simple salads, side dishes, hearty entrees, and baked goods. We've even created coffee drinks and cocktails to round it all out. Don't worry about precision or perfection. Have fun experimenting by trying these ingredients in your everyday favorites like smoothies, salads, and desserts. Once you do, incorporating these items will be easy and effortless—not to mention hugely beneficial to your health. We hope you enjoy reading this book as much as we enjoyed writing it. *Salud!*

# 1 ⌒ PICHUBERRY

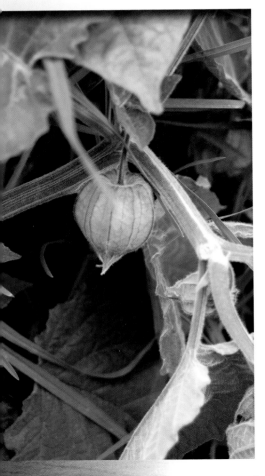

The pichuberry grows wild in the Sacred Valley of the Andes.

## OVERVIEW

**POSSIBLY THE GREATEST SUPERFRUIT** available in the United States, the pichuberry is a small orange fruit the size and shape of a cherry tomato. But don't let its unassuming appearance fool you. This little treasure is bursting with powerful nutrients. And when it comes to taste, the pichuberry explodes with tart yet sweet flavor, like a hybrid of cherry and passionfruit.

This wonder fruit packs a healthy mineral and nutritional composition that surpasses most other conventional and exotic fruits. And that fact is catching the attention of scientists throughout the world. In Peruvian traditional medicine, the pichuberry is used to treat cancer and other diseases like hepatitis, asthma, malaria, and dermatitis.

The pichuberry is rich in vitamins and phenols. In fact, it's packed with vitamin D, an essential vitamin in which most Americans are deficient. The pichuberry also contains withanolides, a rare but special group of antioxidants that have been shown to suppress carcinogens and reduce oxidative stress. Rich in heart-healthy fatty acids, the pichuberry has a remarkably low glycemic index (GI) of 25 (compared to a GI of 50 for blueberries and 53 for the pomegranate). It even contains protein: 1.7 grams in just 3 ounces! And at just 65 calories, it's a diabetes- and weight-loss-friendly fruit.

A distinctive feature of the pichuberry is the papery wrapper or calyx that encloses each individual berry. This protective cover gives the pichuberry a shelf life of about 15 to 20 days in a refrigerated environment.

The pichuberry hails from the highlands of Peru, Chile, and Colombia. Discovered by English settlers, this South American treat became a delicacy in South Africa and parts of Asia and Europe—particularly, France—where it is still relished.

*Truly a culinary treat, the pichuberry brings a unique flavor profile that enhances dishes both savory and sweet. It's a versatile fruit that can be eaten plain or used in everything from breads to salads to desserts. You can add pichuberries to yogurts, oatmeal, waffles, smoothies, and more.*

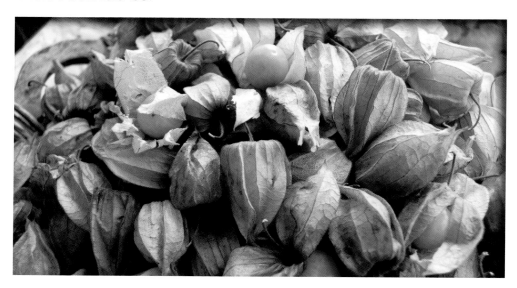

When we visited local farms, we pulled the husk-encased fruits from low bushes and ate them on the spot.

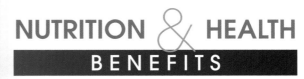

# NUTRITION & HEALTH

## BENEFITS

ANTICANCER

ANTI-INFLAMMATORY

HEART HEALTHY

LOW GLYCEMIC INDEX

SUPPORTS WEIGHT LOSS

Pichuberries are a good source of vitamin E, vitamin A, vitamin P, and the B-complex vitamins $B_1$, $B_6$, and $B_{12}$. By eating only 3 ounces of this power fruit, you'll meet 37 percent of your daily required vitamin A, 13 percent of your required niacin, 18 percent of your recommended vitamin C, and 39 percent of your vitamin D requirement. (Percent daily values are based on a 2,000-calorie diet.)

As many as 77 percent of Americans are vitamin D deficient, which means they lack critical nutrients for healthy bones, happy moods, and optimal immunity. Recent research reveals that a deficit of vitamin D can lead to weight gain. Up until now, we've always been told to get more sunlight in order to take in more vitamin D, but extra sunlight carries the risk of wrinkles and skin cancer. By eating pichuberries, we get plenty of vitamin D without any negative side effects—and they can help us keep weight down by helping to burn fat and keep hunger at bay. Now that's an anti-aging agent!

Pichuberries contain a large group of naturally occurring active chemical compounds called withanolides. There has been a strong link between withanolides and the inhibition of cancer cell growth. In fact, one study showed that withanolides inhibited the formation of new blood vessels that can promote tumor growth, and another study showed that they can even prevent tumor cells from invading healthy ones.

Withanolides help prevent inflammation, linking them to pain relief and managing inflammatory diseases such as arthritis. They also display other significant benefits, including antimicrobial, antitumor, anti-inflammatory, and antibacterial effects.

Pichuberries have a high content of phenolic compounds (aka phenols), which are a natural antioxidant. Vitamin C and phenolic compounds are known to be great free-radical scavengers. Free radicals cause oxidation, which can lead to many chronic diseases.

The whole pichuberry contains oil that is rich in 15 fatty acids, including linoleic acid, an essential oil that cannot be produced by humans.

Pichuberry oil also has high levels of vitamin E, beta-carotene, vitamin $K_1$, and vitamin P, an important flavonoid that helps us absorb vitamin C properly.

The oil extracted from the skin and pulp of the fruit contains high levels of plant sterols. Plant sterols are known to help reduce cholesterol levels, especially the bad cholesterol (LDL).

Pichuberries have a low glycemic index of 25, which makes them a diabetes- and weight-loss-friendly fruit.

We consider pichuberries a powerful anti-aging agent because their vitamin C content and withanoloids help reduce oxidation and inflammation, two conditions that can cause more rapid cellular aging.

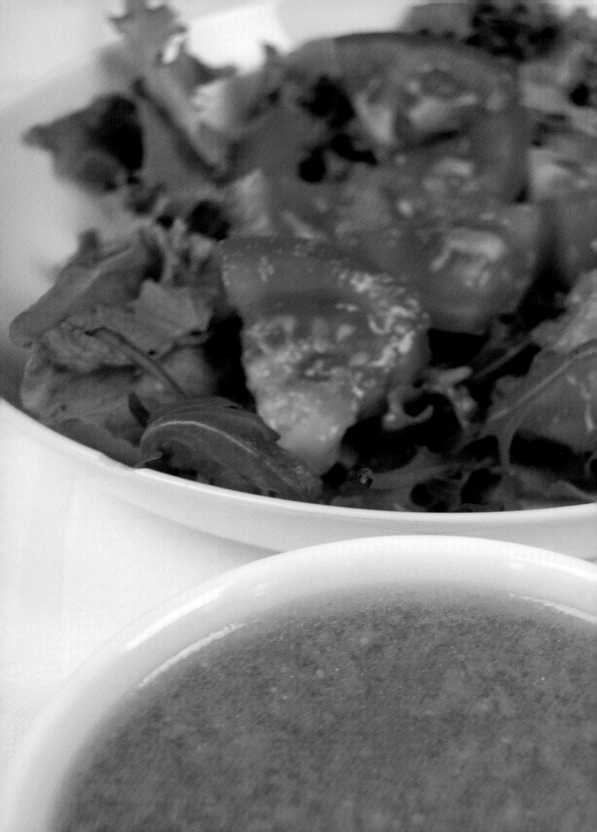

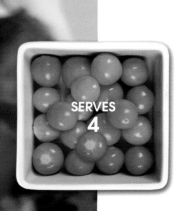

SERVES
4

# PICHUBERRY ORANGE CHAMPAGNE VINAIGRETTE

*Because pichuberries are both tart and sweet, they're a perfect ingredient for salad dressings. Try this one over mixed greens with avocado or baked white fish, like sea bass or cod.*

## Ingredients

3 ounces pichuberries, pureed in the blender

2 ounces orange muscat or regular champagne vinegar

1 tablespoon honey

1 tablespoon lemon juice

2 tablespoons sacha inchi oil

Pinch of salt

## Directions

1. Combine all of the ingredients in a shaker bottle or a blender and thoroughly blend. The vinaigrette will keep in an airtight container for up to a week in the refrigerator.

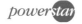 

Per Serving: Kcal 115, Protein 0g, Carb 11g, Fat 7g, Sodium 11mg, Dietary Fiber 0g

Daily Values: Fiber 1%, Vit C 7%, Vit A 8%, Vit D 8%, Calcium 0%, Iron 0%

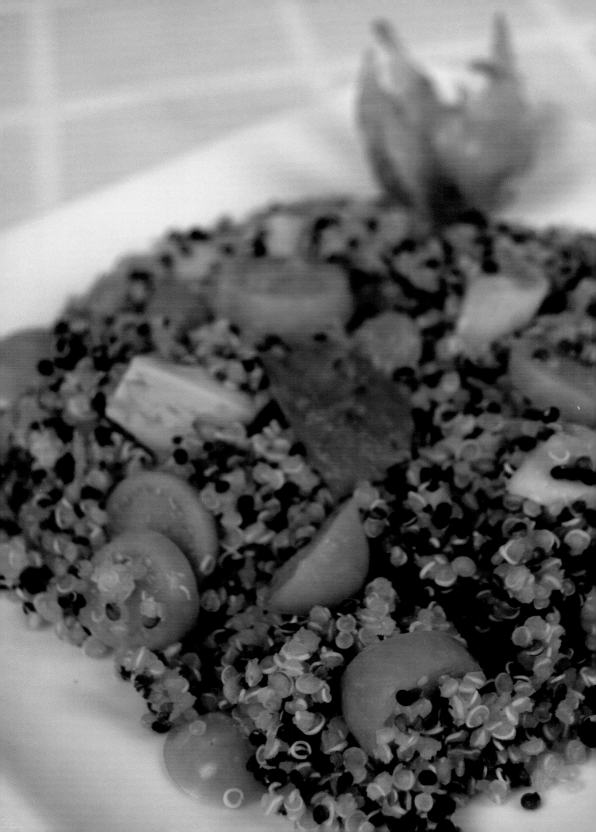

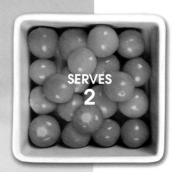

**SERVES 2**

# QUINOA PICHUBERRY SALAD

*Here, textures and fresh flavors meld for a simple yet satisfying summer salad. Try it as an accompaniment to chicken or fish, or dress it up with olives and feta for a heartier stand-alone dish.*

## Ingredients

1 cup cooked red or white quinoa
1 small avocado, diced
3 ounces pichuberries, quartered
Juice of one orange
Salt to taste

## Directions

1. Combine the quinoa, avocado, and pichuberries in a bowl and squeeze the fresh orange juice on top. Season with salt and gently fold together.

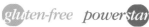 *gluten-free* **powerstar** *vegan*

**Per Serving:** Kcal 269, Protein 6g, Carb 36g, Fat 12g, Sodium 33mg, Dietary Fiber 8g
**Daily Values:** Fiber 31%, Vit C 52%, Vit A 19%, Vit D 17%, Calcium 3%, Iron 10%

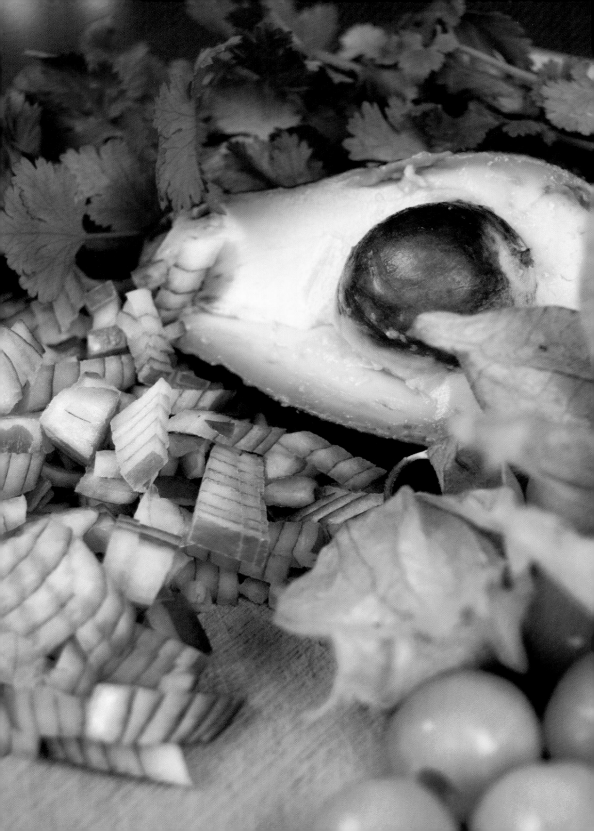

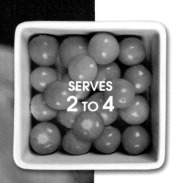

# PICHUBERRY GUACAMOLE

*Add pichuberries to a summer classic for an unexpected hint of fruit flavor. We love this over fish tacos as well as with blue corn chips.*

**SERVES 2 TO 4**

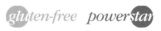

PICHUBERRY RECIPES

## Ingredients

1 avocado, pitted and cut into smaller pieces
3 ounces pichuberries; 2 ounces crushed and 1 ounce quartered
2 tablespoons chopped cilantro
2 tablespoons diced red onion
Salt to taste

## Directions

1. Place the avocado pieces in a bowl and then add the remaining ingredients. Mix thoroughly until the guacamole reaches the desired chunky consistency. Enjoy!

*gluten-free*  *powerstar*  *vegan*

Per Serving: Kcal 101, Protein 2g, Carb 10g, Fat 7g, Sodium 23mg, Dietary Fiber 3g
Daily Values: Fiber 14%, Vit C 14%, Vit A 16%, Vit D 15%, Calcium 1%, Iron 2%

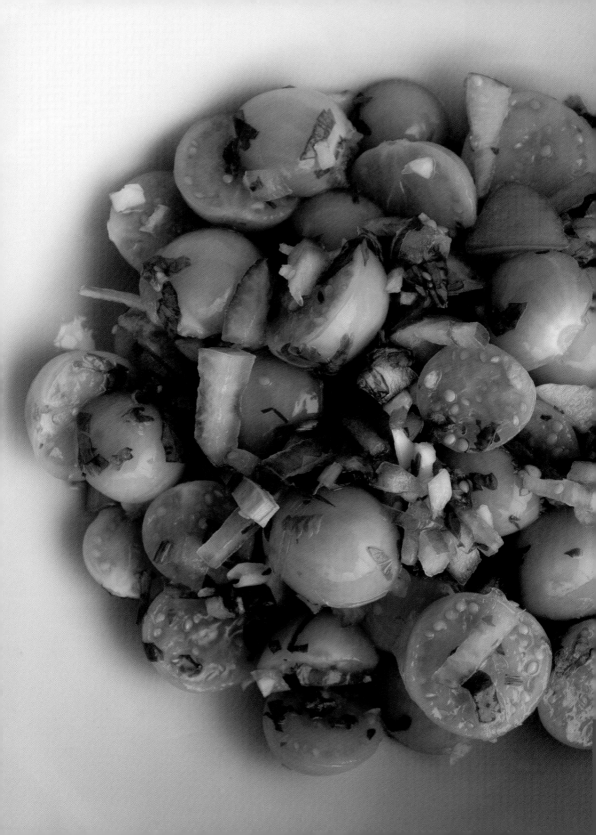

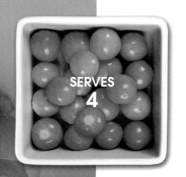

SERVES
4

# PICHUBERRY SALSA

*Pichuberries make a great stand-in for a traditional tomato salsa. Try this variation over pork, chicken, or fish.*

## Ingredients

1 cup diced pichuberries
Juice of 2 limes (about ¼ cup juice)
2 teaspoons honey
1 heaping tablespoon chopped cilantro
1 small clove garlic, finely minced
2 tablespoons finely chopped red onion or sweet onion

## Directions

1. Combine all of the ingredients in a small bowl and refrigerate until serving time. The flavors are best if the salsa is refrigerated for 4 hours or overnight.

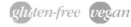 *gluten-free*  *vegan*

**Per Serving:** Kcal 39, Protein 1g, Carb 10g, Fat 0g, Sodium 18mg, Dietary Fiber 1g
**Daily Values:** Fiber 2%, Vit C 15%, Vit A 13%, Vit D 13%, Calcium 1%, Iron 0%

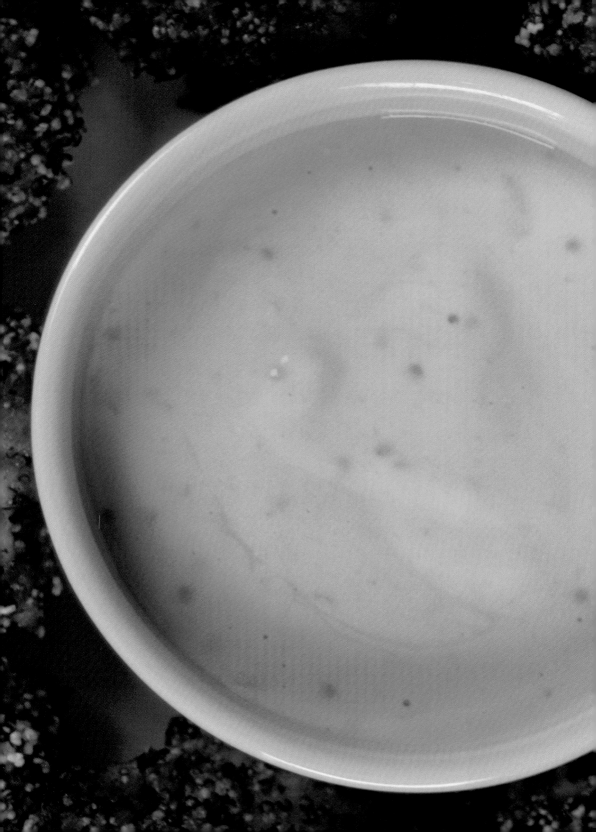

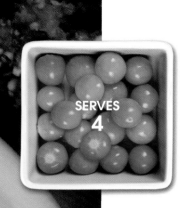

**SERVES 4**

# PICHUBERRY HONEY MUSTARD DIPPING SAUCE

*We wanted to make a kid-friendly sauce for homemade chicken tenders or carrots. The result was this zesty mix, which is a smart alternative to store-bought dips, with a great flavor that will please all ages.*

## Ingredients

¾ cup Greek yogurt
2 tablespoons honey
2 tablespoons yellow mustard
¼ cup pureed pichuberries

## Directions

 In a small bowl, whisk all of the ingredients together until blended. Refrigerate for 1 hour.

 *gluten-free* 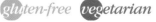 *vegetarian*

**Per Serving:** Kcal 69, Protein 1g, Carb 12g, Fat 0g, Sodium 91mg, Dietary Fiber 0g
**Daily Values:** Fiber 2%, Vit C 2%, Vit A 4%, Vit D 4%, Calcium 5%, Iron 1%

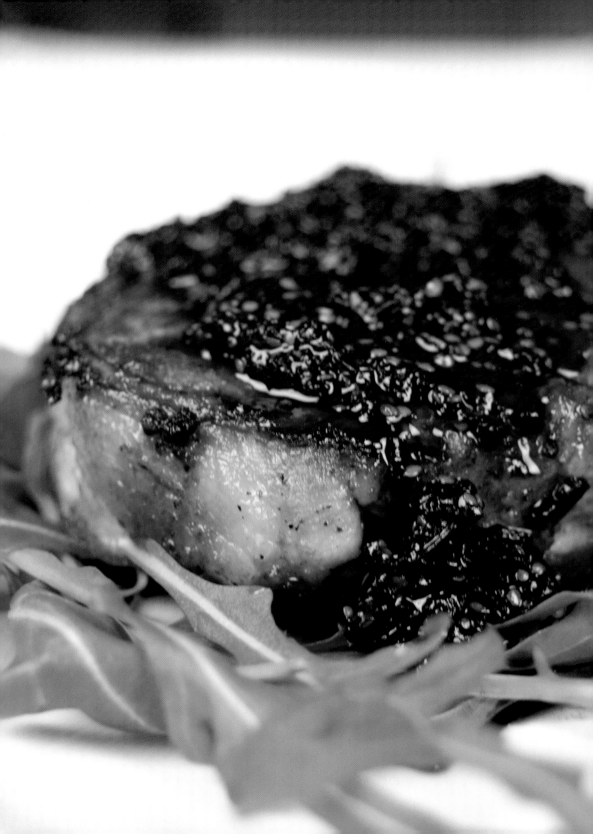

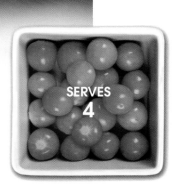

**SERVES 4**

# BALSAMIC PICHUBERRY REDUCTION

*This may be the simplest recipe in the book, but it's also one of the most flavorful. Try this piquant reduction over pork loin or white fish for an elegant entrée.*

## Ingredients

¾ cup balsamic vinegar

1 cup pureed pichuberries

1 tablespoon agave nectar

## Directions

1. Combine all of the ingredients in a saucepan and bring to a boil. Reduce to simmer until the sauce thickens, stirring occasionally, roughly 15 minutes.

*glu*ten-free

**Per Serving:** Kcal 86, Protein 1g, Carb 18g, Fat 0g, Sodium 33mg, Dietary Fiber 0g
**Daily Values:** Fiber 2%, Vit C 8%, Vit A 16%, Vit D 17%, Calcium 2%, Iron 2%

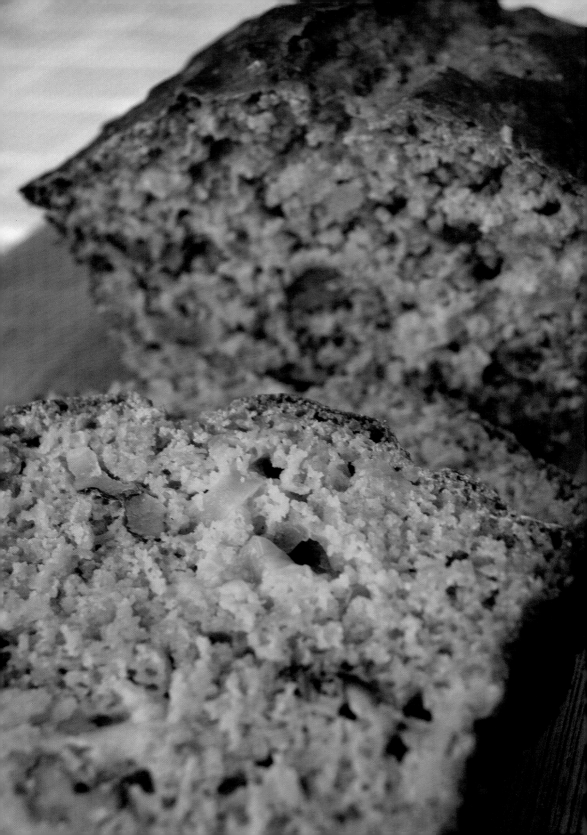

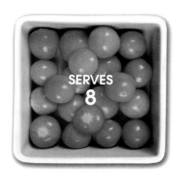

**SERVES 8**

# HEARTY QUINOA PICHUBERRY BREAD

*We wanted to make a tasty, gluten-free, fruit-and-nut bread packed with flavor, but minus the added sugar. Here, the fruit and agave act as sweeteners, and the result is a dense, moist loaf that's great for breakfast or an afternoon snack. The yogurt and quinoa add protein, so it's a perfectly balanced nutritional food.*

## Ingredients

1½ cups fresh pichuberries, pureed

4 tablespoons plain nonfat
   Greek yogurt

½ cup agave nectar

1 teaspoon vanilla extract

2 eggs

1 teaspoon baking soda

1 teaspoon baking powder

1 teaspoon salt

2 cups oat flour

1 cup cooked quinoa

½ cup fresh pichuberries,
   sliced in halves

½ cup chopped walnuts

## Directions

1. Preheat the oven to 350 degrees F.

2. Thoroughly combine the pichuberry puree, Greek yogurt, agave nectar, vanilla extract, and eggs in a large bowl. Gently fold in the baking soda, baking powder, salt, oat flour, quinoa, pichuberry slices, and the walnuts.

3. Spray a 9-inch loaf pan with nonstick spray. Add the batter and place in the oven on the middle rack. Bake for 70 minutes or until golden brown and a toothpick placed into the center comes out clean.

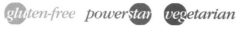 *gluten-free* **powerstar** *vegetarian*

**Per Serving:** Kcal 281, Protein 9g, Carb 44g, Fat 9g, Sodium 491mg, Dietary Fiber 4g
**Daily Values:** Fiber 16%, Vit C 8%, Vit A 17%, Vit D 17%, Calcium 6%, Iron 11%

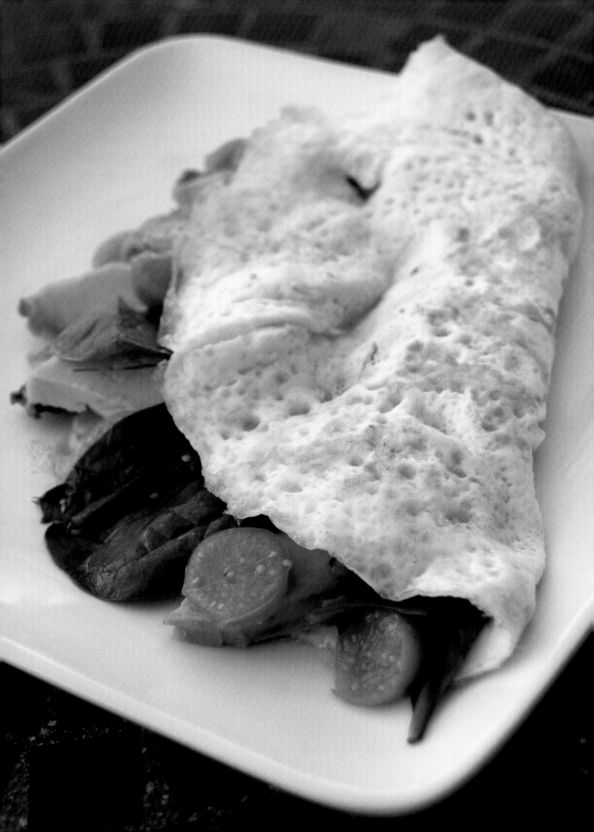

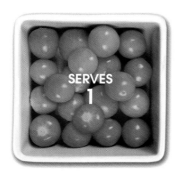

**SERVES
1**

# PICHUBERRY
# AVOCADO OMELET

*We've become so enamored of the pichuberry,
in all its versatility, that we started using it in
some pretty unexpected ways. One morning,
Manuel was craving avocado and pichuberry
together so he devised this omelet, which is
now a favorite in his breakfast rotation. Using
egg whites instead of regular eggs makes for an
even lighter, but equally energy-boosting, start
to the day.*

## Ingredients

½ cup egg whites

Salt and pepper to taste

6 pichuberries, sliced in halves

½ avocado, thinly sliced lengthwise

½ cup fresh spinach

## Directions

**1** Heat a nonstick pan over low-medium heat and spray it with nonstick
cooking spray.

**2** Season the egg whites with salt and pepper. Pour them into the pan
and evenly distribute. Cover and cook until the egg whites are no longer
runny, roughly 2 minutes.

**3** Top half of the egg white with the pichuberry slices, avocado, and
spinach, and fold the other half over to cover it. Wait about 30 seconds
to a minute until the spinach wilts a bit, and then use a spatula to gently
lift the omelet onto a plate.

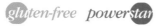 *gluten-free powerstar vegetarian*

**Per Serving:** Kcal 208, Protein 16g, Carb 15g, Fat 11g, Sodium 246mg, Dietary Fiber 5g
**Daily Values:** Fiber 22%, Vit C 26%, Vit A 50%, Vit D 21%, Calcium 4%, Iron 6%

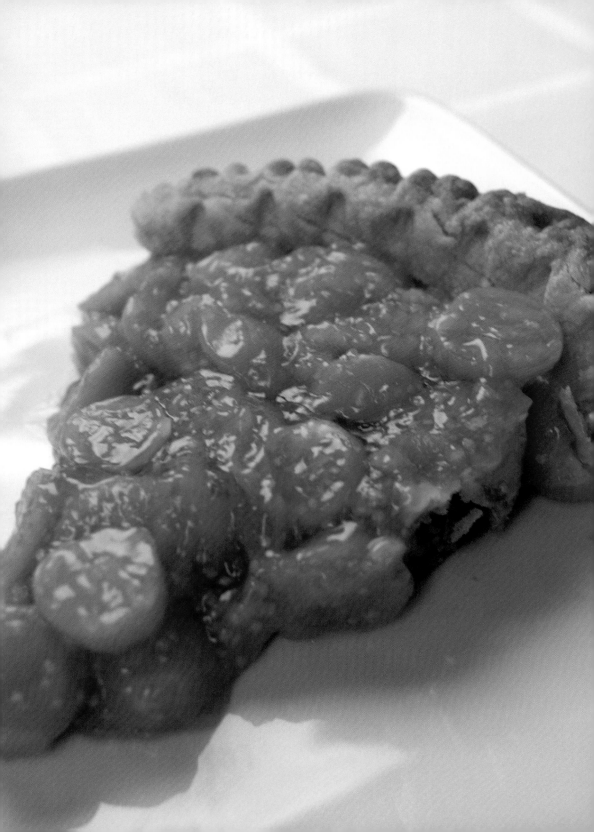

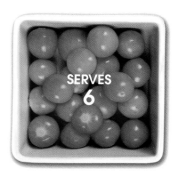

SERVES
6

# PICHUBERRY PIE

*A very versatile fruit that lends itself to savory and piquant dishes as well as sweet ones, the pichuberry holds its own as the star attraction in a classic dessert like this simple, open-faced pie.*

## Ingredients

9-inch baked pie crust

3 cups fresh pichuberries, sliced in halves

½ cup water

2 tablespoons cornstarch

2 tablespoons water

½ cup sugar

2 teaspoons fresh lemon juice

Pinch of salt

## Directions

1   Preheat the oven to 400 degrees F.

2   Measure 1 cup of the pichuberries. Place them in a medium saucepan with ½ cup water. Cover and bring to a boil.

3   In a small bowl, whisk together the cornstarch and the 2 tablespoons of water.

4   When the pichuberries and water have come to a boil, lower the heat and simmer, stirring constantly for 3 to 4 minutes, or until the pichuberries start to burst. Stirring constantly, add the cornstarch mixture, sugar, lemon juice, and salt. Simmer for a minute or until the mixture becomes translucent. Immediately remove it from the heat and quickly fold in the remaining 2 cups of pichuberries.

5   Spoon the mixture into the prepared pie shell and allow it to sit at room temperature for at least 2 hours before serving.

*vegetarian*

**Per Serving:** Kcal 271, Protein 3g, Carb 42g, Fat 10g, Sodium 190mg, Dietary Fiber 2g
**Daily Values:** Fiber 7%, Vit C 13%, Vit A 25%, Vit D 26%, Calcium 1%, Iron 5%

# PICHUBERRY STRAWBERRY GALETTE

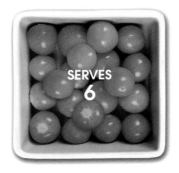

SERVES 6

*For a variation on the traditional pie, try this elegant galette. It's easy to whip up and the pretty folded edges make it an attractive option to share with guests.*

## Ingredients

¼ cup all-purpose flour, plus extra flour for rolling

1 teaspoon salt

1 teaspoon sugar

½ cup (1 stick) cold unsalted butter, cut into pieces

2 to 8 tablespoons ice water

1 cup pichuberries, sliced in halves

1 cup strawberries, stemmed and quartered

Milk to brush dough (optional)

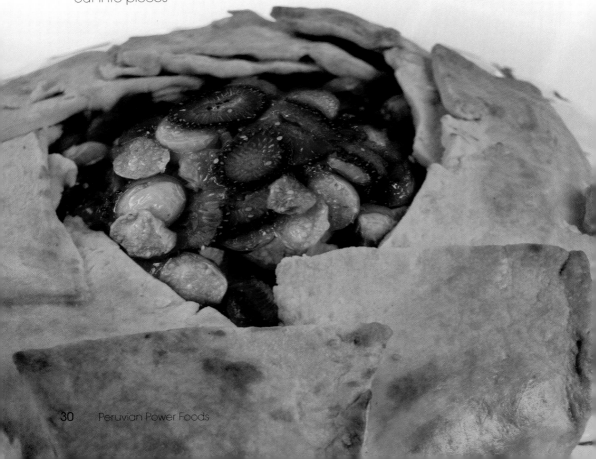

## Directions

**1** Preheat the oven to 350 degrees F.

**2** In a food processor or standing mixer, mix the flour, salt, and sugar. Add the butter and mix until it resembles a coarse meal, with a few pea-size pieces of butter remaining. Sprinkle with 1 tablespoon ice water at a time, just until it binds. (Only use as much ice water as required to form the dough; otherwise it may become too wet and sticky.)

**3** Press the dough into a 1-inch disk and wrap it in plastic cling wrap. Refrigerate until firm, at least 1 hour (or up to 3 days).

**4** Flour a work surface and roll the dough with a floured rolling pin out to a 14-inch round.

**5** Pile the sliced fruit in the center of the dough round, leaving 2 to 3 inches of dough uncovered around the perimeter.

**6** Using a sharp knife, make 2-inch slits into the dough perimeter, toward the center, every 3 inches around the circle. (Imagine marking where every other numeral might sit around a clock face). These slits create panels that you'll fold up to encase the fruit.

**7** Lift one 3–inch panel and fold it up over the fruit, and then fold the next one up over the first, pinching the seam closed where the two panels overlap. The goal is to make a dough container for the fruit by folding the flaps up over the fruit. The better you're able to seal the seams, the more successful your end product will be. If your seams are not properly sealed, you'll notice fruit juices seeping out during the baking, and this can cause the galette to stick to the pan.

**8** Once the panels are sealed, use two spatulas to lift the galette onto a parchment-lined cookie sheet or silicon baking liner. Brush the dough with milk if you want a golden crust.

**9** Bake until the dough is golden brown, approximately 20 to 30 minutes.

*vegetarian*

**Per Serving:** Kcal 180, Protein 1g, Carb 10g, Fat 16g, Sodium 402mg, Dietary Fiber 1g
**Daily Values:** Fiber 3%, Vit C 28%, Vit A 18%, Vit D 11%, Calcium 1%, Iron 2%

PICHUBERRY RECIPES

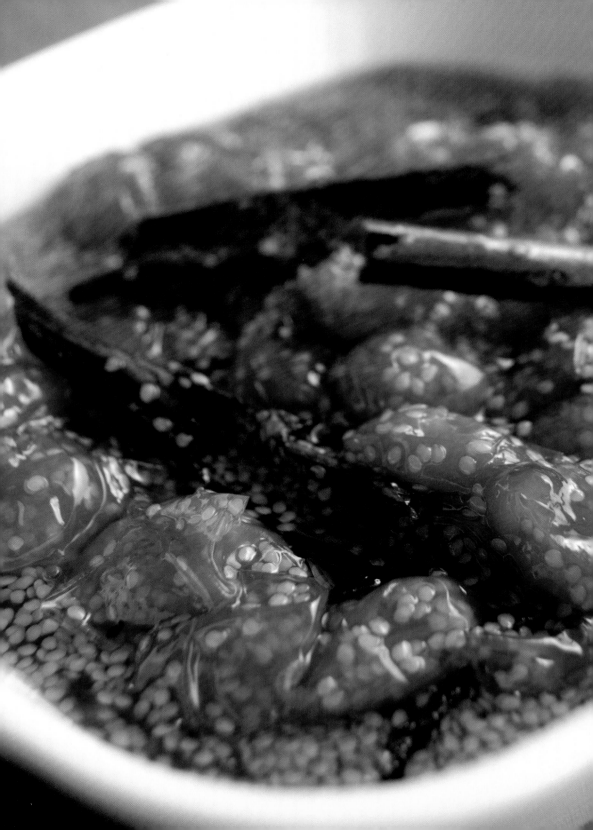

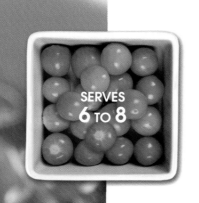

**SERVES
6 TO 8**

# PICHUBERRY MARMALADE

*This recipe comes from a dear family friend, Norma. While we were visiting Lima and playing with pichuberry recipes, she threw together this simple, wonderful marmalade.*

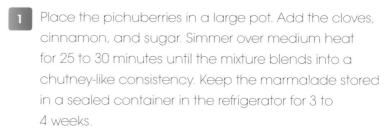

## Ingredients

2½ cups pichuberries, sliced in halves
4 cloves
1 cinnamon stick
½ cup sugar

## Directions

1  Place the pichuberries in a large pot. Add the cloves, cinnamon, and sugar. Simmer over medium heat for 25 to 30 minutes until the mixture blends into a chutney-like consistency. Keep the marmalade stored in a sealed container in the refrigerator for 3 to 4 weeks.

**Per Serving:** Kcal 87, Protein 1g, Carb 21g, Fat 0g, Sodium 24mg, Dietary Fiber 1g
**Daily Values:** Fiber 2%, Vit C 9%, Vit A 18%, Vit D 19%, Calcium 1%, Iron 0%

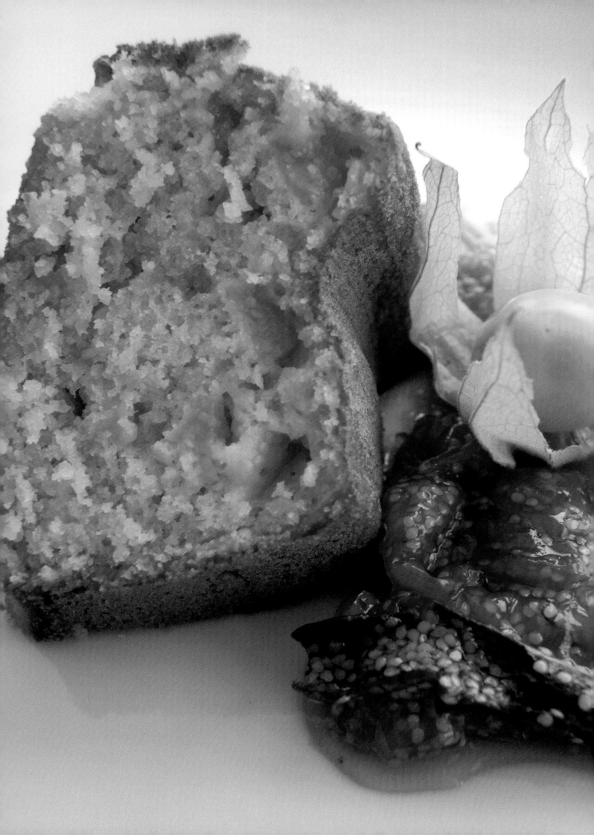

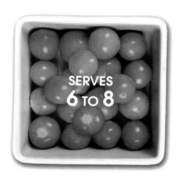

SERVES
**6 TO 8**

# PICHUBERRY CAKE

*Manuel has fond memories of eating an orange-infused cake when he was growing up. This version replaces the citrus flavor with pichuberries for a tart and sweet take on a family classic.*

## Ingredients

1 cup sugar

3 ounces butter

2 cups all-purpose flour

2 teaspoons baking powder

3 eggs

2 cups pureed pichuberries, blended until liquid

½ cup pichuberries, sliced in halves

## Directions

1. Preheat the oven to 350 degrees F.

2. Beat the sugar and butter until creamy. Mix in the flour and baking powder, and then incorporate the eggs one by one while beating.

3. Pour in the pichuberry liquid and mix until fully integrated into the batter. With a spatula, gently fold in the remaining pichuberries.

4. Grease a ring/bundt pan with butter and sprinkle it with flour. Add the batter to the pan and bake for 25 to 30 minutes or until a toothpick inserted near the center comes out clean.

*vegetarian*

**Per Serving:** Kcal 391, Protein 7g, Carb 64g, Fat 12g, Sodium 126mg, Dietary Fiber 1g
**Daily Values:** Fiber 6%, Vit C 0%, Vit A 8%, Vit D 4%, Calcium 8%, Iron 12%

# 2 ⌒ MACA

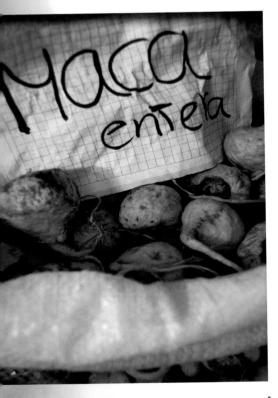

At the height of their empire, Incan warriors consumed maca before battle, believing it would give them strength. However, legend has it they were prohibited from taking it after conquering a city in order to protect the women from their strong sexual impulses. Maca is still regarded as a potent sexual stimulant today. When we visited the open market in Cuzco and asked a few elderly women what maca is good for, they giggled and said, "The bedroom."

## OVERVIEW

**MACA IS A NATIVE** Peruvian plant that grows in the tropical Andes, dating back to approximately 3800 BC. Resembling a small rough stone the size of a walnut, maca is a powerful energy booster that can be used to increase libido, treat erectile dysfunction, improve concentration, and enhance workout performance by increasing strength and endurance. It's referred to by some as "Peruvian ginseng" for its similarly stimulating qualities.

A good source of calcium, maca is a wonderful option for women seeking nutritional supplements to support bone health. In every 10 grams or 2 teaspoons of maca, there are 25 mg of calcium. Rich in iron and protein, maca is also a perfect solution for vegetarians and vegans looking for meat-free alternatives. Maca is also a good source of vitamin C; two teaspoons has about 28 mg, which is 30 to 37 percent of the daily requirement for men and women, respectively. This potent concentration boosts the immune system, and works to prevent cardiovascular disease and eye disease.

Because maca is a starch, it can be difficult to digest in its raw form. Today, you can purchase raw maca powder or a gelatinized version, which helps break down the starch content and makes it easier to digest and absorb. The type you purchase is really a matter of personal preference—both deliver the powerful benefits explained below.

Maca hails from the Andes, land of the Inca, where it is still a powerful and popular food source today. In order to start feeling the natural energy (which doesn't carry the same side effects as caffeine), you'll need to take it consistently for at least a week. Try adding a tablespoon to a smoothie each morning to enjoy it the way Peruvians do.

*Unlike most of the other superfoods derived from fruits and seeds, maca carries a distinctly bitter taste, so it's best to use it in recipes that mask the flavor. We've had great results pairing it with cacao, cinnamon, banana, and other foods with pronounced flavors. While some of the power foods shared in this book burst with great taste that you'll want to showcase, this is one that's best used in smoothies, power bars, desserts, and other dishes that meld ingredients.*

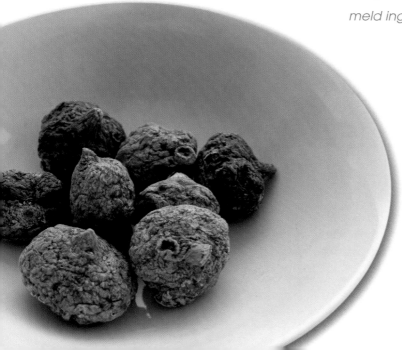

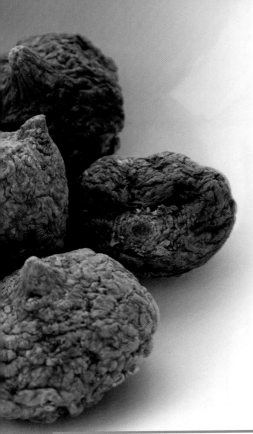

# NUTRITION & HEALTH
## BENEFITS

AIDS ERECTILE DYSFUNCTION

BOOSTS LIBIDO

CONTROLS ANEMIA

DECREASES MENSTRUAL AND
MENOPAUSAL SYMPTOMS

DETOXIFIES

ENHANCES ATHLETIC PERFORMANCE

IMPROVES FERTILITY

INCREASES ENERGY

Rich in essential amino acids; calcium; copper; iodine; iron; manganese; phosphorus; protein; vitamins $B_6$, vitamin $B_{12}$, $B_1$, $B_2$, and E; and zinc.

Dried maca powder contains more than 10 percent protein and 7 essential amino acids.

With high amounts of calcium and iron, maca meets the increased need for essential minerals in women.

Maca has a positive effect on energy and mood, making it a perfect pre-workout supplement. It can even support continued exercise after extended effort because studies show it increases glucose in the blood stream after a prolonged fast.

Maca balances hormones and increases fertility.

Maca contains vitamin C and iron—two essential nutrients that help prevent anemia. One tablespoon of maca provides 8 percent of the daily requirement of iron; since vitamin C increases the absorption of iron, maca is a perfect solution for women during the menstrual cycle.

Studies suggest that maca boosts energy and immunity because of its amino acid profile and mineral content. Maca contains phytochemicals and flavanols that can scavenge various free radicals (the bodily bad guys that, left unchecked, can lead to disease).

A greater intake of maca significantly increases semen volume, total sperm count, motile sperm count, and sperm motility. Maca has also been shown to improve male sexual performance in men with mild erectile dysfunction.

Maca may reduce anxiety and heighten sexual desire for both men and women. Studies suggest that by activating key endocrine glands, maca increases energy, vitality, and libido.

Maca protects cells from the toxicity that comes from chronic inflammation and oxidative stress.

Maca is considered an anti-aging aid because it increases libido and energy and helps to protect and strengthen bones. By balancing hormones like testosterone, progesterone, and estrogen, maca has the power to help forestall the hormonal changes of aging.

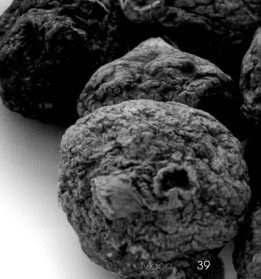

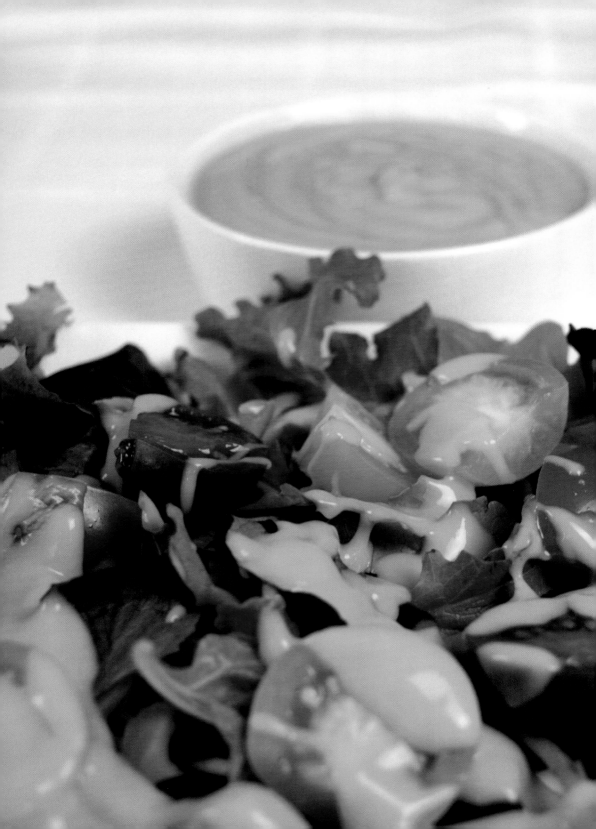

**SERVES
8**

# CREAMY AVOCADO
# MACA DRESSING

*Looking for an alternative to the traditional
vinaigrette? This maca-avocado dressing brings
creamy texture and a citrus kick to any bowl of
greens or grains.*

## Ingredients

1 avocado
2 tablespoons agave nectar
¼ cup fresh lime juice
2 tablespoons maca
1 cup orange juice

## Directions

1  Combine all of the ingredients in a bowl and blend
until smooth with a hand mixer. A food processor is fine
to use as well.

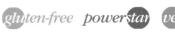 *gluten-free*  **power**  *vegan*

**Per Serving:** Kcal 68, Protein 1g, Carb 11g, Fat 3g, Sodium 2mg, Dietary Fiber 1g
**Daily Values:** Fiber 6%, Vit C 33%, Vit A 2%, Vit D 0%, Calcium 1%, Iron 1%

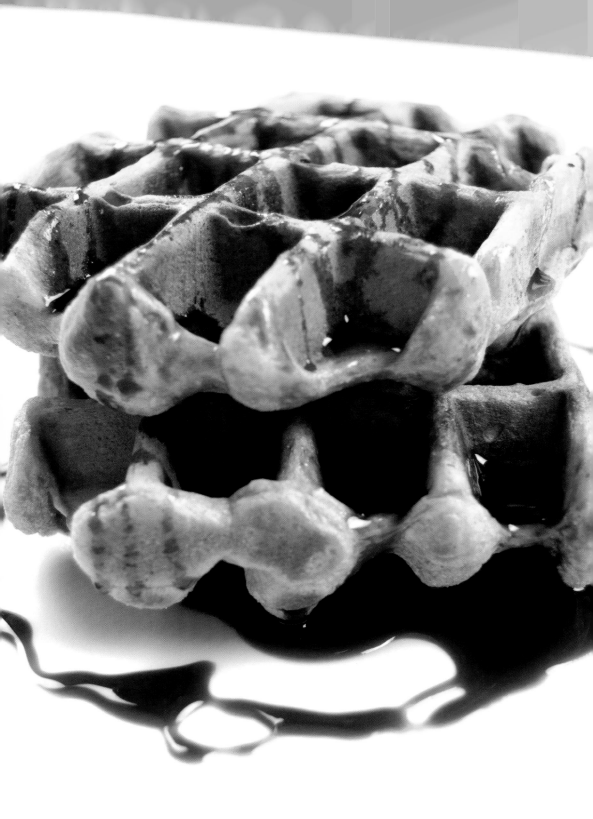

# MACA WAFFLES

**SERVES 2**

*Since maca is such a great booster for strength, energy, and endurance, it makes sense to build breakfast around it for a powerful start to the day. These waffles are just the thing before a workout or a long day in the office.*

## Ingredients

1 cup all-purpose flour

2 teaspoons baking powder

2 tablespoons maca

1 dash salt

1 egg

¾ cup milk

¼ cup unsweetened applesauce

1 teaspoon vanilla extract

3 tablespoons coarsely chopped walnuts

## Directions

1. In a large bowl, sift together the flour, baking powder, maca, and salt.

2. In a medium bowl, combine the egg, milk, applesauce, and vanilla extract.

3. Make a small well in the middle of the dry ingredients and add the liquid mixture into it. Gently combine all of the ingredients until the batter is just smooth.

4. Pour the batter into a preheated waffle maker and cook until golden brown. Serve with the chopped walnuts.

**NOTE:** *If you prefer, you can make pancakes with this recipe.*

vegetarian

**Per Serving:** Kcal 433, Protein 17g, Carb 67g, Fat 11g, Sodium 373mg, Dietary Fiber 4g
**Daily Values:** Fiber 16%, Vit C 3%, Vit A 6%, Vit D 14%, Calcium 38%, Iron 25%

**MACA RECIPES**

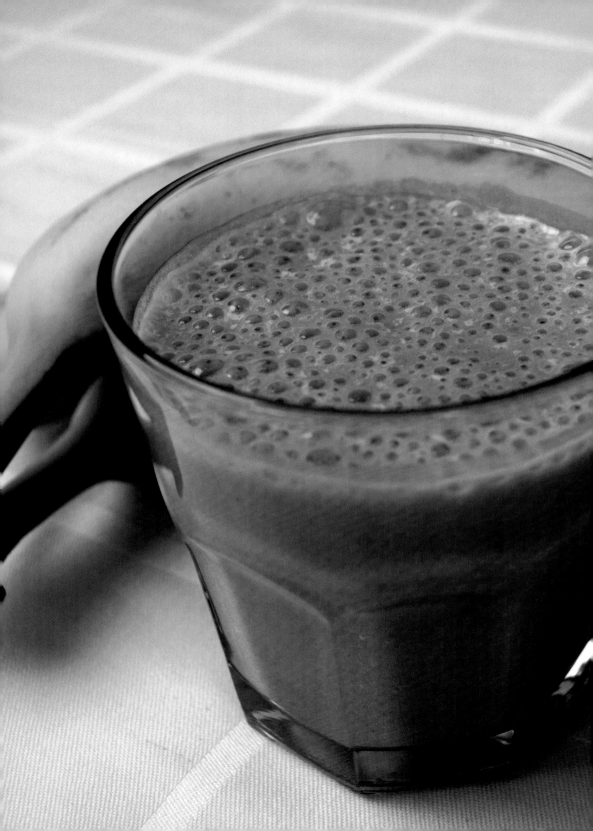

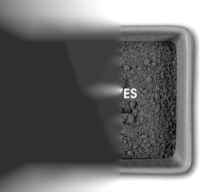

# MACA BANANA LUCUMA SMOOTHIE

*This smoothie couldn't be easier, more delicious, or more effective in delivering key nutrients. With a combination of maca and lucuma, you get the dual benefits of extra energy and powerful antioxidants. With a slightly maple flavor, lucuma (see page 170) is a nice complement to the banana.*

(see page 170)

## Ingredients

1 banana
1 cup milk of choice
1 tablespoon maca
1 tablespoon lucuma

## Directions

 Combine all of the ingredients in a blender and mix until smooth.

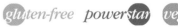 gluten-free  powerstar   vegan

**Per Serving:** Kcal 303, Protein 12g, Carb 59g, Fat 3g, Sodium 114mg, Dietary Fiber 4g
**Daily Values:** Fiber 16%, Vit C 19%, Vit A 11%, Vit D 32%, Calcium 32%, Iron 6%

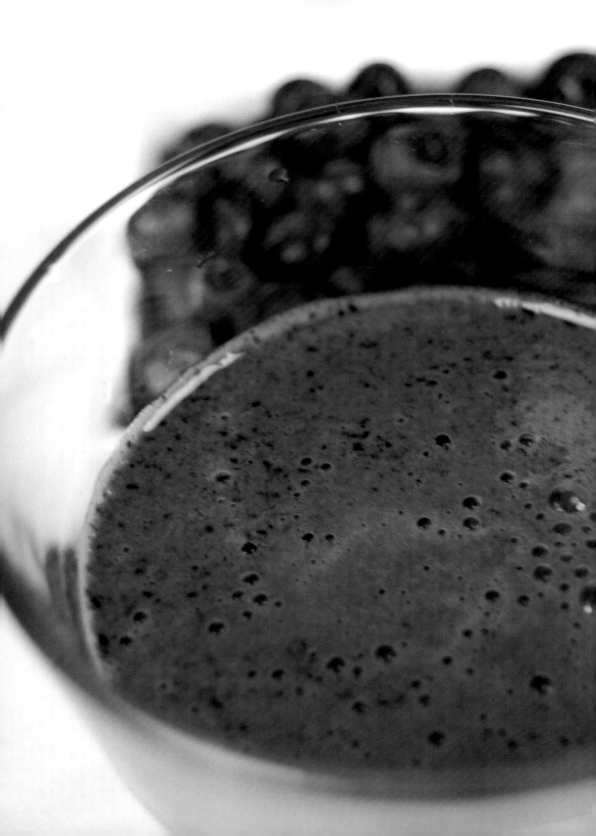

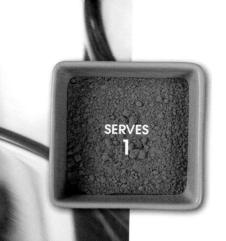

**SERVES
1**

# CACAO BLUEBERRY
# MACA SHAKE

*Berries go beautifully with chocolate flavors, so
this pairing is a rich and delicious treat. You'll
get the energy-boosting power of maca plus
the double antioxidant power of blueberries
and cacao.*

## Ingredients

1 cup milk of choice
1 tablespoon maca
1 tablespoon cacao
¾ cup blueberries, frozen or fresh

## Directions

Combine all of the ingredients in a blender and mix
until smooth.

**MACA RECIPES**

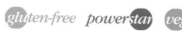

*gluten-free* **power**star *vegan*

**Per Serving:** Kcal 259, Protein 12g, Carb 46g, Fat 3g, Sodium 108mg, Dietary Fiber 6g
**Daily Values:** Fiber 25%, Vit C 18%, Vit A 11%, Vit D 32%, Calcium 30%, Iron 9%

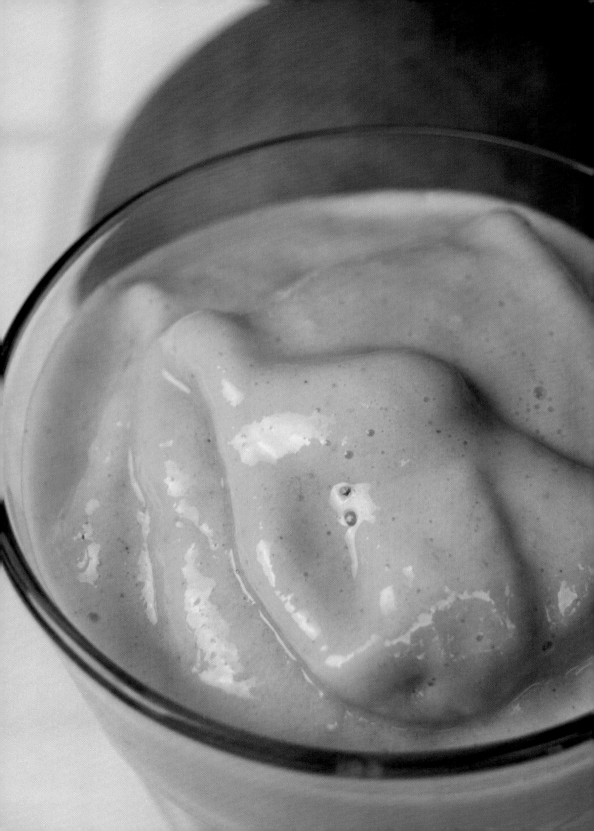

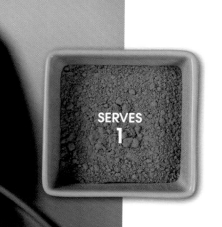

# MACA MANGO COOLER

*Somewhere between a refreshing frosty milk treat and a yogurt drink like Indian lassi, this whipped blend is perfect for a hot summer day.*

## Ingredients

1 cup frozen mango chunks
1 cup milk of choice
1 teaspoon agave nectar
1 tablespoon maca

## Directions

1  Combine all of the ingredients in a blender and mix until smooth. Enjoy with a spoon.

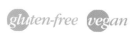

gluten-free  vegan

**Per Serving:** Kcal 266, Protein 10g, Carb 53g, Fat 3g, Sodium 111mg, Dietary Fiber 4g
**Daily Values:** Fiber 16%, Vit C 78%, Vit A 35%, Vit D 32%, Calcium 33%, Iron 4%

**MACA RECIPES**

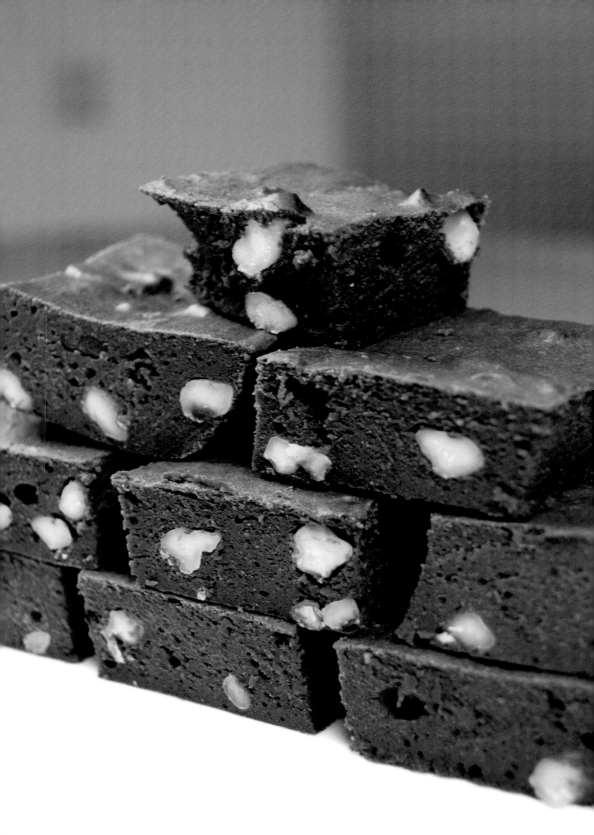

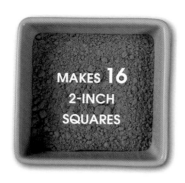

**MAKES 16 2-INCH SQUARES**

# MACA FUDGE BROWNIES

*Here's another wonderful way to mask maca's bitter flavor while enjoying its energy-boosting power. Combining maca with antioxidant-rich cacao, these brownies are a hit because they deliver the benefits of maca and the taste of a decadent dessert.*

## Ingredients

1 cup all-purpose flour
½ cup cacao powder
¼ teaspoon salt
4 tablespoons maca
2 ounces dark chocolate, chopped
½ cup agave

2 tablespoons coconut oil
⅓ cup 1% milk
1 teaspoon vanilla extract
2 large egg yolks
1 egg
½ cup applesauce

## Directions

1. Preheat the oven to 350 degrees F.

2. Combine the flour, cacao, salt, and maca in a large bowl. Stir with a whisk.

3. In a microwave-safe bowl, microwave the chocolate at high heat for 30 seconds, stirring at the 15-second mark. Add the agave and coconut oil, stir, and heat for an additional 15 seconds, or until the mixture is smooth. Set aside to cool slightly.

4. Once the chocolate mixture has cooled, add the milk, vanilla, egg yolks, egg, and applesauce. Stir with a whisk to combine.

5. Add the chocolate mixture to the flour mixture, stirring until just combined. Pour the batter into a greased 8-inch-square baking dish. Bake on the middle rack for 20 minutes or until a wooden toothpick inserted in the center comes out clean.

*powerstar* *vegetarian*

**Per Serving:** Kcal 135, Protein 3g, Carb 21g, Fat 4g, Sodium 44mg, Dietary Fiber 2g
**Daily Values:** Fiber 7%, Vit C 1%, Vit A 1%, Vit D 2%, Calcium 2%, Iron 5%

# 3 ⌢ CACAO

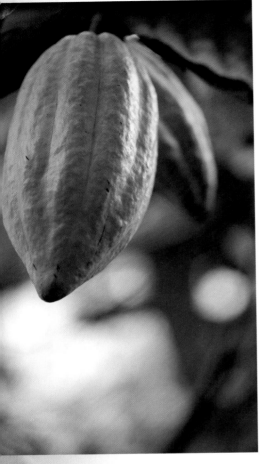

Cacao was cultivated over 3,000 years ago by Incans in Peru. They called it "the food of the gods" because they believed it worthy enough to be a divine offering. Once discovered by the New World, it was still highly prized and designated as a drink reserved for nobles.

## OVERVIEW

**CACAO IS A SMALL BROWN BEAN** resembling a coffee bean, which is processed to make common chocolate. It is sold in nibs, powders, and bars. While many forms of chocolate are diluted with sugars and fillers, the finest chocolates in the world retain a high percentage of cacao—not only for its smooth, rich, decadent taste, but also for its miraculous health and anti-aging benefits. When we eat chocolate in its raw form, we derive the most benefits. Today, most chocolate undergoes extreme processing and loses its natural nutrients. In its natural state, however, chocolate can help with weight loss, increased energy, heart health, and more.

Cacao is loaded with vitamins and antioxidants that make it a natural multi-vitamin. Raw cacao is rich in antioxidants, essential minerals, vitamins, and natural mood-enhancing nutrients called theobromine and phenylethylamine. The latter is a super low-potency antidepressant that works like the body's dopamine and adrenaline. Phenylethylamine is known as the "pleasure chemical" because it's secreted by people in love; no wonder people are head over heels about chocolate! Cacao can increase the amount of serotonin your brain produces, which can create a balancing effect and sense of well-being. And of course, all of these effects explain why so many women mysteriously crave chocolate when suffering from PMS! Chocolate is produced by liquefying cacao nibs or seeds without the shell, to create what is known as chocolate liquor. It's then pressed into powder or bars using a weighted press. The darker and less processed the chocolate you choose, the more cacao included, and hence, the more powerful the health benefits.

*Obviously, the primary culinary use for cacao is to make chocolate. From there, cacao can be used in almost any recipe that might call for chocolate nibs, powder, or liquor. The best thing is, it imparts the rich, satisfying taste of high-quality chocolate while delivering a strong dose of anti-aging antioxidants—something that can't be said for more diluted and processed forms of chocolate.*

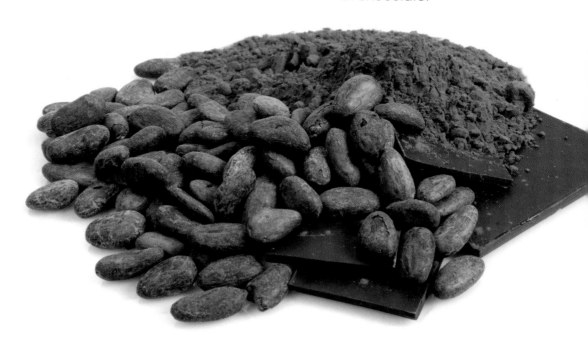

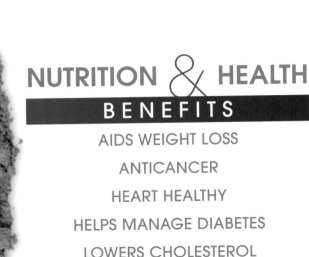

# NUTRITION & HEALTH
## BENEFITS

AIDS WEIGHT LOSS

ANTICANCER

HEART HEALTHY

HELPS MANAGE DIABETES

LOWERS CHOLESTEROL

STRENGTHENS IMMUNE SYSTEM

SUPPORTS BRAIN HEALTH

Cacao is rich in essential vitamins A, $B_1$, $B_2$, $B_3$, C, E, and pantothenic acid. It also contains a high amount of polyphenols. In addition, cacao beans are loaded with essential minerals like calcium, copper, iron, magnesium, manganese, potassium, and zinc.

Cacao has more antioxidants than black tea, green tea, or red wine, which means it has the antioxidant power equivalent to vitamin C. It can help treat inflammation and potentially help fight cancer, inflammatory diseases, and cardiovascular disease.

Cacao is a natural appetite suppressant, so it can help reduce food cravings and aid in weight loss.

Cacao beans contain iron, omega-6 fatty acids, and theobromine, which play an important role in heart health and brain function.

Cacao polyphenols have been proven to protect against nerve cell injury and inflammation; thus, cacao may play a role in protecting the brain from normal degeneration or even from neurodegenerative diseases.

Antioxidants, including polyphenols, catechins, and epicatechins, help to fight off free radicals, which, left unchecked, can cause many chronic diseases.

Cacao has been shown to decrease blood pressure, both systolic and diastolic, and to increase vasodilation of the blood vessels. It also decreases total cholesterol and LDL (bad) cholesterol and increases HDL (good) cholesterol.

Numerous studies show that cacao phenolics lower insulin resistance and sensitivity, so it may be useful in managing diabetes.

Cacao flavanols are scientifically proven to help support healthy circulation by helping your arteries stay supple. Cacao has also been shown to build resistance to oxidative stress, which can cause inflammation and atherosclerosis. For this reason, cacao is a phenomenal anti-aging agent.

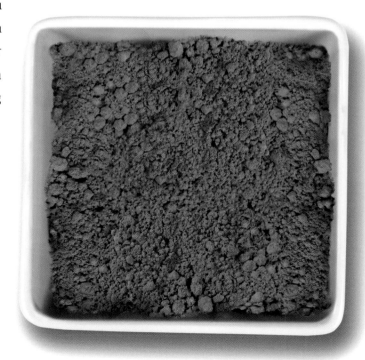

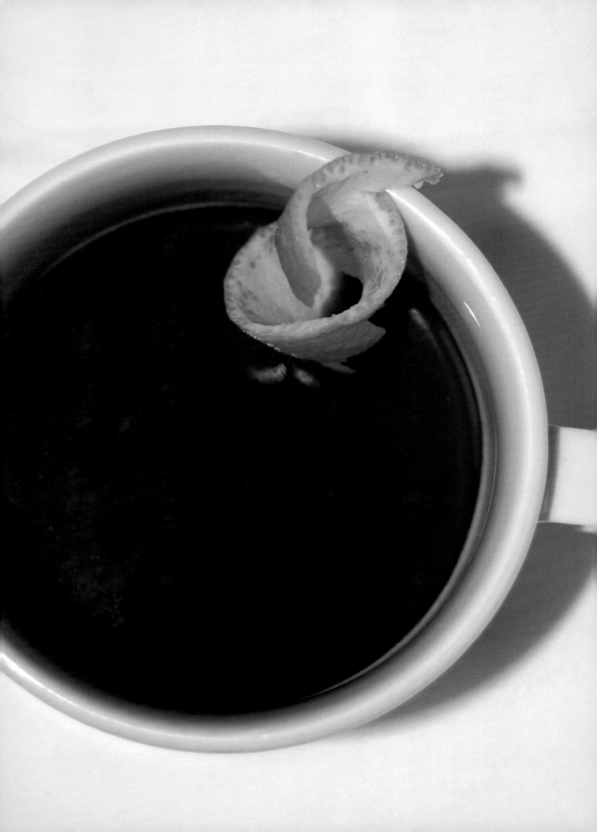

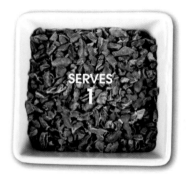

# CUZCO COFFEE

*This divine concoction was inspired by Café Ayllu, a longtime local favorite in Cuzco, where the coffee beans are roasted with orange peel and onion skins then brewed up into a thick, hot chocolate blend. We created our own version, skipping the onion skins.*

## Ingredients

1 shot espresso

1 tablespoon cacao powder

1 teaspoon agave

1 orange

1 shot of pisco (optional)

## Directions

1. Brew 1 shot of espresso or very strong black coffee. Stir in the cacao and agave until blended thoroughly. Pour the mixture into an espresso demitasse cup.

2. Using a potato peeler or a paring knife, cut a 3-inch by 1-inch curl from the outer skin of an orange, taking care not to include the white pith. Run a match or lighter on the underside of the skin to release the orange oils. Then curl the orange skin around your finger to create a decorative curl for a garnish, either in or on the side of the coffee cup. You can also add a spritz of orange for extra citrus flavor.

OPTIONAL: *Want to take it up a notch? Add a shot of pisco and this café becomes an after-dinner drink.*

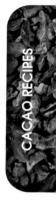

CACAO RECIPES

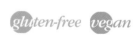 *gluten-free* *vegan*

**Per Serving:** Kcal 111, Protein 2g, Carb 25g, Fat 1g, Sodium 6mg, Dietary Fiber 5g
**Daily Values:** Fiber 19%, Vit C 116%, Vit A 6%, Vit D 0%, Calcium 6%, Iron 4%

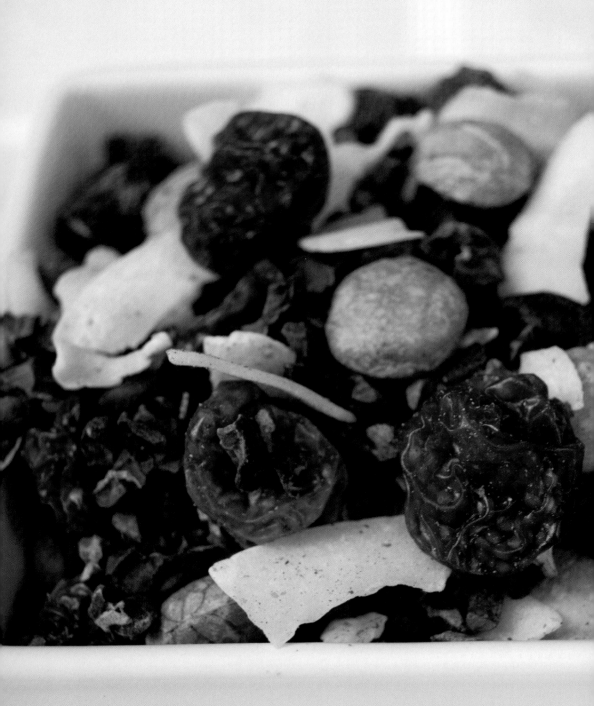

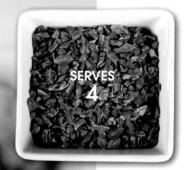

**SERVES 4**

# POWER TRAIL MIX

*When it came to strength and endurance, the Incas knew what was up. This combination of potent power foods is just the boost you need for a strenuous workout or a stressful day at work.*

## Ingredients

¼ cup cacao nibs
¼ cup dried pichuberries
¼ cup dried unsweetened coconut flakes
¼ cup roasted sacha inchi seeds

## Directions

1. Combine all of the ingredients in a bowl and mix them together. Store in an airtight container at room temperature for up to a week.

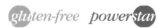  
*gluten-free   powerstar   vegan*

**CACAO RECIPES**

**Per Serving:** Kcal 235, Protein 2g, Carb 9g, Fat 22g, Sodium 9mg, Dietary Fiber 4g
**Daily Values:** Fiber 18%, Vit C 1%, Vit A 12%, Vit D 0%, Calcium 1%, Iron 4%

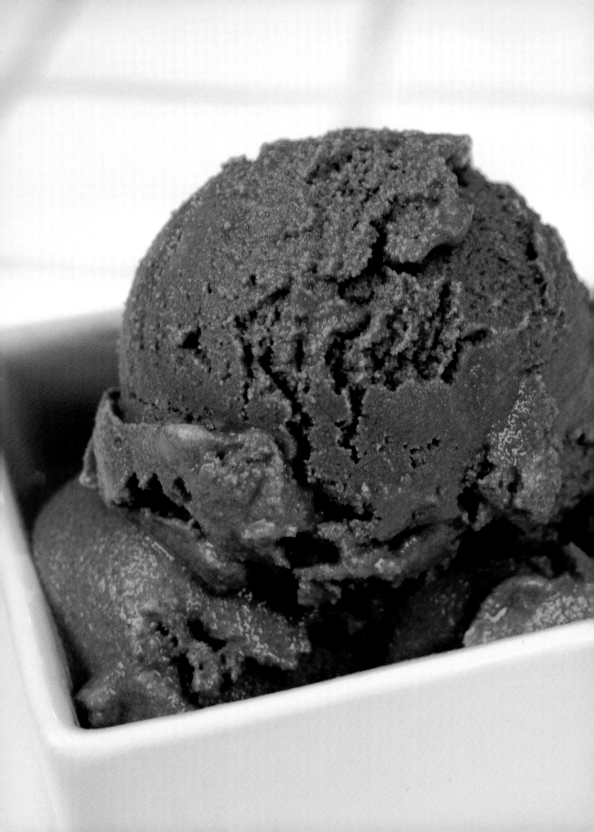

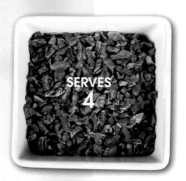

**SERVES 4**

# DARK CHOCOLATE FROZEN YOGURT

*Here, cacao brings deep, dark flavor to healthy Greek yogurt for a dessert treat you can feel great about.*

## Ingredients

1 cup 1% milk
½ cup agave nectar
1 cup sifted cacao powder
1 teaspoon vanilla extract
1½ cups 2% Greek yogurt

## Directions

**1** Combine all of the ingredients in a bowl and whisk until evenly combined. Cover and refrigerate for 1 to 2 hours. Then prepare according to your ice-cream maker manufacturer's instructions.

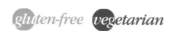 gluten-free vegetarian

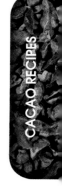

CACAO RECIPES

**Per Serving:** Kcal 316, Protein 15g, Carb 53g, Fat 5g, Sodium 62mg, Dietary Fiber 6g
**Daily Values:** Fiber 26%, Vit C 0%, Vit A 2%, Vit D 8%, Calcium 20%, Iron 13%

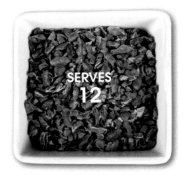

SERVES
12

# DRUNKEN CACAO TRUFFLES

*If you had any doubt that power foods can be utterly addictive and delicious, you only need to try one of these boozy truffles. We could not believe how rich and luscious they tasted.*

## Ingredients

½ cup pisco
½ cup dried pichuberries
3½ ounces (100 grams) dark
   chocolate (73% dark)

¼ cup coconut cream
1 tablespoon agave
2 tablespoons cacao powder

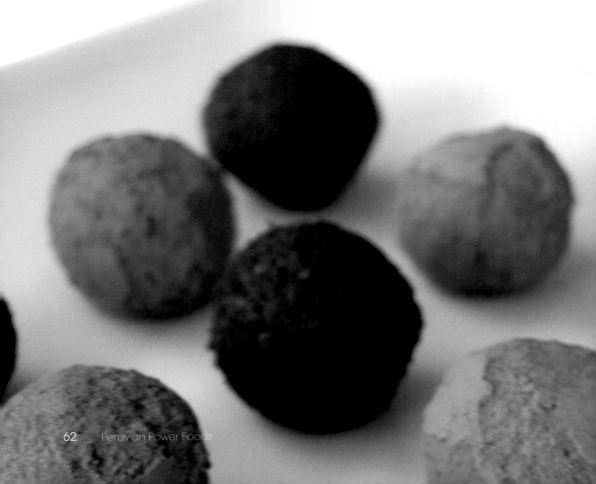

## Directions

**1** In a medium bowl, soak the dried pichuberries in pisco for at least 6 hours at room temperature. This can also be done overnight.

**2** Once the pichuberries have soaked and softened, remove them from the pisco and set the pisco aside. In a food processor, blend the pichuberries to create a paste.

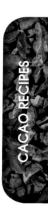

**3** Add 2 to 3 inches of water to a pot. Bring the water to a simmer. Keeping the heat very low, place the bowl of chocolate on top of the simmering water. Make sure the bowl does not touch the water by leaving 1 to 2 inches between the water and bowl. The steam from the simmering water is sufficient to melt the chocolate. Note: Avoid spilling water into the chocolate.

**4** Stir the chocolate constantly to ensure even melting. By keeping the heat very low and constantly stirring, you can melt the chocolate without overheating it. When you see the chocolate is almost melted, remove the bowl from the simmering pot of water and stir the chocolate until smooth and shiny.

**5** In a separate saucepan, warm the coconut cream and 3 ounces of the pichuberry paste until thoroughly combined. Add the mixture to the melted chocolate. Add the agave and cacao powder. Gently fold in all of the ingredients until thoroughly combined.

**6** Allow the mixture to cool. Then, using your hands, roll the mixture into individual 1½-inch truffles. Refrigerate the truffles in an airtight container for up to 1 week.

*gluten-free* *vegan*

**Per Serving:** Kcal 104, Protein 1g, Carb 10g, Fat 5g, Sodium 5mg, Dietary Fiber 2g
**Daily Values:** Fiber 8%, Vit C 1%, Vit A 8%, Vit D 0%, Calcium 0%, Iron 2%

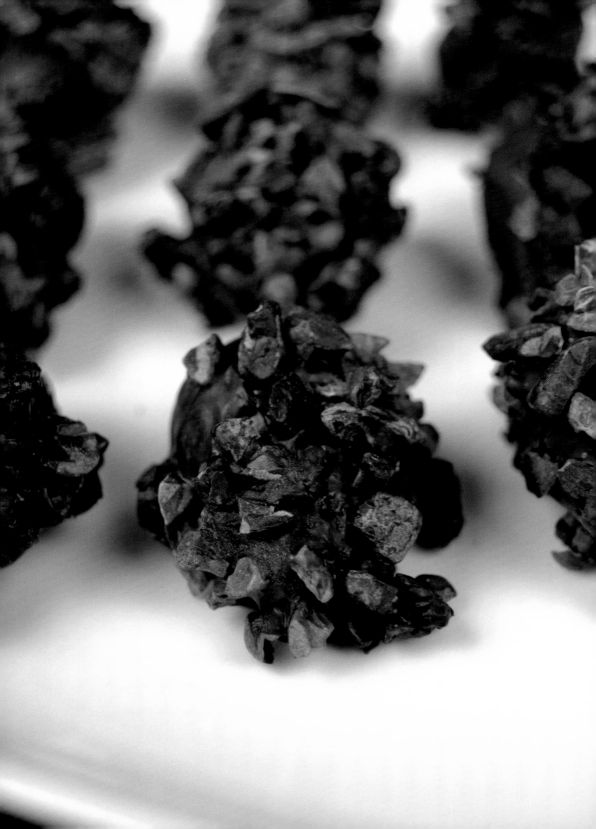

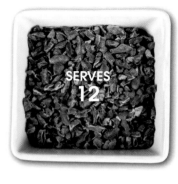

# DARK CHOCOLATE FIGS WITH CACAO

**SERVES 12**

*Chocolate and fruit are a classic flavor combination, and this easy-to-assemble recipe makes an impressive truffle with sophisticated flavor.*

## Ingredients

½ bar (50g) dark chocolate
  (73% dark)

12 dried figs
½ cup to 1 cup cacao nibs

## Directions

1. Chop the chocolate into even pieces to make it easier to melt. Place in a stainless steel bowl.

2. Add 2 to 3 inches of water to a pot. Bring the water to a simmer. Keeping the heat very low, place the bowl of chocolate on top of the simmering water. Make sure the bowl does not touch the water by leaving 1 to 2 inches between the water and bowl. The steam from the simmering water is sufficient to melt the chocolate. Note: Avoid spilling water into the chocolate.

3. Stir the chocolate constantly to ensure even melting. By keeping the heat very low and constantly stirring, you can melt the chocolate without overheating it. When you see the chocolate is almost melted, remove the bowl from the simmering pot of water and stir the chocolate until smooth and shiny.

4. Dip each fig into the melted dark chocolate, covering the fig completely. Place the figs on a sheet of parchment or wax paper. Sprinkle with the cacao nibs.

5. Allow the chocolate-covered figs to harden for about 30 minutes in the refrigerator and enjoy.

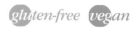

*gluten-free* *vegan*

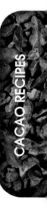

**CACAO RECIPES**

**Per Serving:** Kcal 67, Protein 1g, Carb 9g, Fat 4g, Sodium 0mg, Dietary Fiber 0g
**Daily Values:** Fiber 8.4%, Vit C 29%, Vit A 0%, Vit D 0%, Calcium 0%, Iron 2%

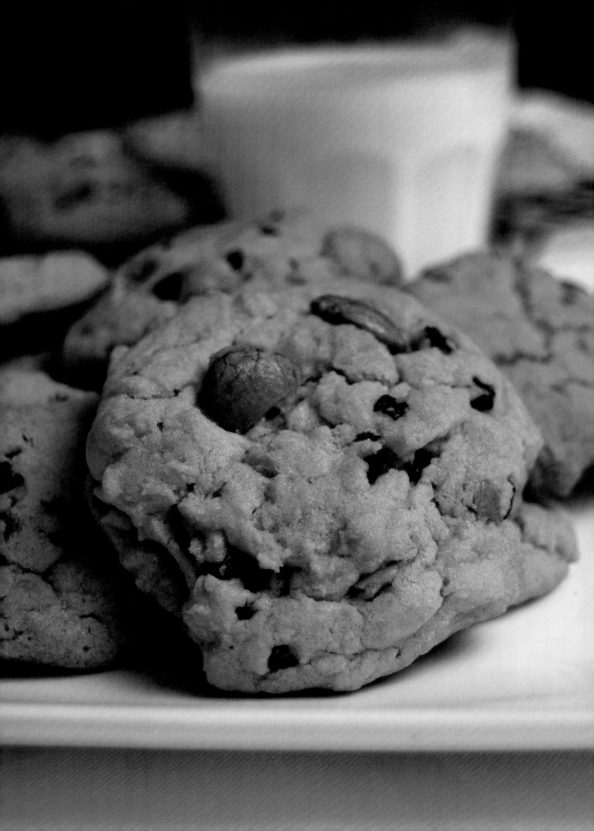

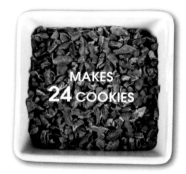

**MAKES 24 COOKIES**

# CACAO CHIP COOKIES WITH ROASTED SACHA INCHI SEEDS

*This is our take on the traditional chocolate chip cookie. Just replace the chocolate with cacao nibs and the nuts with sacha inchi seeds, and the classic kid treat becomes an antioxidant powerhouse!*

## Ingredients

2¼ cups all-purpose flour
1 teaspoon baking soda
¼ teaspoon salt
1 cup packed brown sugar
¾ cup granulated sugar
½ cup butter, softened

1 teaspoon vanilla extract
2 large egg whites
½ cup cacao nibs
½ cup roasted sacha inchi seeds,
   coarsely chopped

## Directions

1. Preheat the oven to 350 degrees F.

2. In a large bowl, combine the flour, baking soda, and salt. Stir with a whisk.

3. In a separate bowl, combine the sugars and butter. Beat with a mixer at medium speed until well incorporated. Add the vanilla and egg whites. Beat for an additional minute.

4. Add the sugar mixture to the flour mixture and beat until blended. Gently fold in the cacao nibs and sacha inchi seeds.

5. Lightly coat a cookie sheet with cooking spray, and spoon 1 tablespoon of batter onto it at a time, keeping each cookie an inch or two apart.

6. Bake for 13 to 15 minutes, or until golden brown.

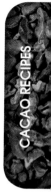

**CACAO RECIPES**

 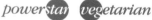
*powerstar* *vegetarian*

**Per Serving:** Kcal 175, Protein 3g, Carb 26g, Fat 7g, Sodium 80mg, Dietary Fiber 2g
**Daily Values:** Fiber 6%, Vit C 0%, Vit A 2%, Vit D 1%, Calcium 1%, Iron 4%

# 4 ☞ KIWICHA

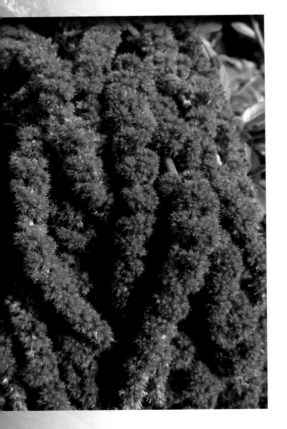

## OVERVIEW

**KIWICHA IS JUST ANOTHER NAME** for amaranth. Sometimes referred to as mini-quinoa, kiwicha is considered a wonder grain because its seeds contain impressive amounts of protein from concentrated amino acids.

Kiwicha is a strong antioxidant, anti-cancer, and anticholesterol compound whose healthful properties offer myriad benefits. A recent report suggests that plant sterols found in kiwicha oil can reduce serum cholesterol levels of the "bad kind" (LDL cholesterol) as well as total cholesterol. These plant sterols also appear to support the health of cell membranes, which may be a benefit for people with high blood pressure.

The kiwicha plant grows in the highlands of Peru, as well as in Bolivia, Ecuador, and Argentina. The "grains" of kiwicha are tiny and poppy-seed-sized, and each plant can produce as many as 100,000 seeds.

Perhaps the most fun food featured in our book, kiwicha is a seed that, while tiny, can be popped into a fluffy kernel like a miniature version of popcorn. Once popped, it becomes a perfect base for all kinds of tasty snacks and dishes. While we were in Cuzco, we noticed that many street vendors were selling popped kiwicha balls sweetened with dates or yacon.

Kiwicha has been cultivated by people living in the Andes for more than 4,000 years. It was a popular staple during the Incan empire, but soon after it was abandoned in favor of other grains. Today, we are rediscovering the wonders of this tiny, health-packed seed.

*In its raw form, kiwicha is an incredibly small seed, but we were delighted to learn that it can be popped just like popcorn, yielding mini white kernels that can be used in energy bars or as the base for breakfast cereals. The trick is popping it quickly and keeping the pan moving so it fluffs up without burning. Once you master this technique, kiwicha is a fun ingredient to have in your repertoire.*

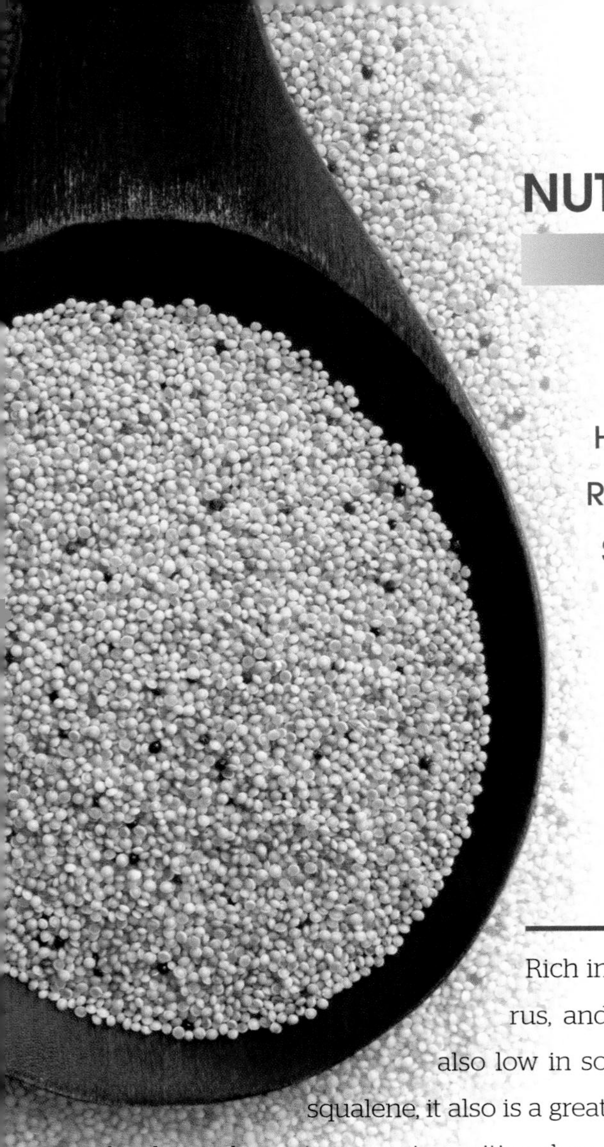

# NUTRITION & HEALTH
## BENEFITS

GOOD PROTEIN SOURCE

HEART HEALTHY

HELPS LOWER CHOLESTEROL

REGULATES BLOOD PRESSURE

SUPPORTS IMMUNE SYSTEM

Rich in iron, magnesium, manganese, phosphorus, and soluble and insoluble fiber, kiwicha is also low in sodium. Loaded with phytochemicals like squalene, it also is a great source of natural antioxidants. Squalene has been shown to promote positive changes in the immune systems and to prevent cancer.

In numerous studies, kiwicha has been proven to reduce LDL or "bad cholesterol."

Kiwicha contains fiber and it's a complete source of protein, meaning it contains all 9 essential amino acids. This is a great option for vegetarians and vegans seeking plant-based protein sources.

With a balanced carbohydrate and protein content and no gluten, kiwicha is perfect for people with Celiac disease and gluten sensitivity and intolerance.

Kiwicha has been shown to be an ACE inhibitor. ACE is an enzyme that stimulates an increase in blood pressure. This suggests kiwicha's possible role in reducing hypertension.

For its benefits to the heart, blood pressure, and cholesterol levels, we classify kiwicha as a wonderful anti-aging agent.

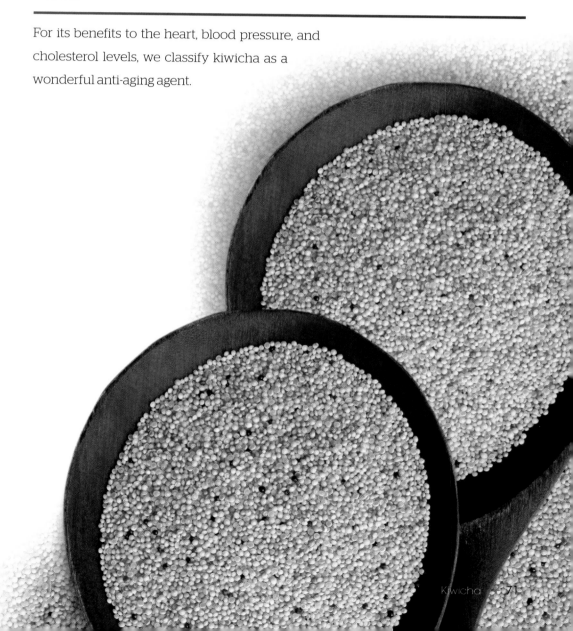

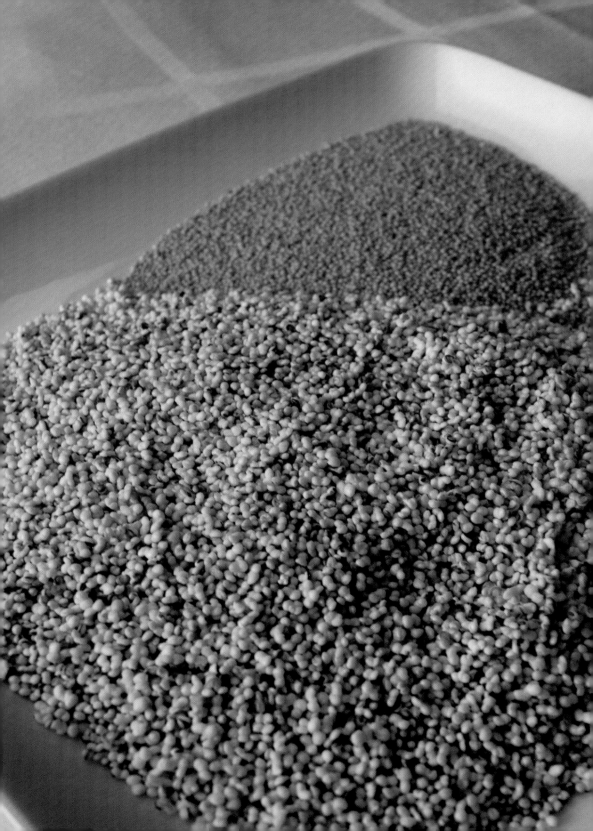

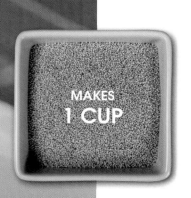

# POPPED KIWICHA

**MAKES**
**1 CUP**

*Imagine our delight when we learned we could pop this fine grain into fluffy little kernels like micropopcorn. Once you do, you can snack on it plain, or use it as the base for the other recipes in this section. Three tablespoons of raw kiwicha makes 1 cup popped.*

## Ingredients

3 tablespoons dry/raw kiwicha

## Directions

**1**  Heat a medium frying pan over high heat until the entire surface is extremely hot. Add 1 tablespoon of kiwicha and evenly distribute it in the pan. No oil is needed. Cover the pan with a glass lid and allow the kiwicha to "pop" until white, roughly 30 seconds, making sure to move the pan over the heat to ensure even heat distribution. When popped, remove the kiwicha from the heat and pan immediately.

**2**  Repeat step 1 until the desired amount of kiwicha is popped. It may take a round or two of trial and error to get the heat, movement of the pan, and the timing just right, but you'll get the hang of it in no time, and then popping kiwicha will be fun as well as practical.

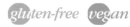  *gluten-free* *vegan*

Per Serving: Kcal 344, Protein 15g, Carb 63g, Fat 5g, Sodium 116mg, Dietary Fiber 6g
Daily Values: Fiber 26%, Vit C 20%, Vit A 11%, Vit D 32%, Calcium 35%, Iron 18%

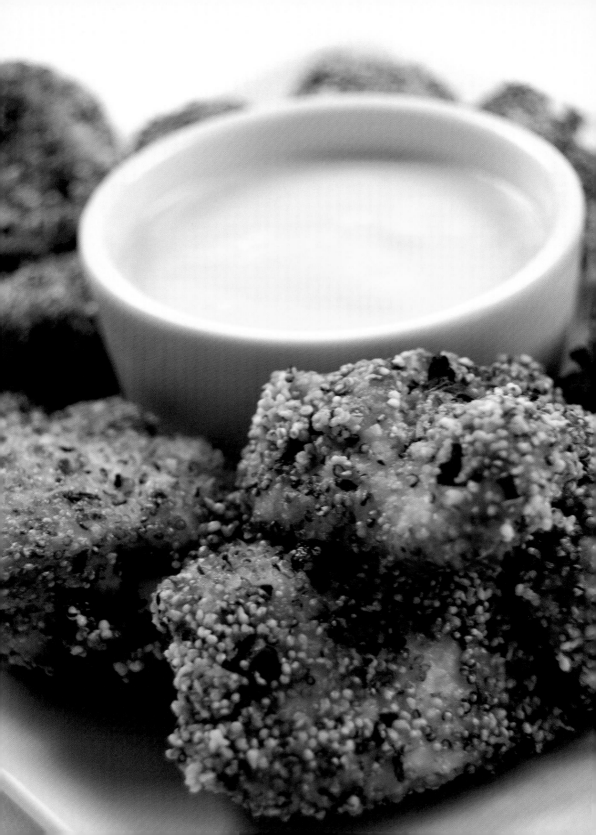

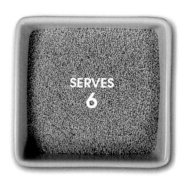

# KIWICHA CHICKEN NUGGETS

**SERVES 6**

*While we were researching kiwicha and other power foods in Cuzco, we noticed that local restaurants used the grain to "bread" meat. That's when we realized kiwicha makes a great gluten-free option for coating chicken, as in these kid-friendly nuggets, or even for a more adult-style baked chicken dish.*

## Ingredients

3 boneless skinless chicken breasts

1 cup popped kiwicha
    (3 tablespoons raw)

½ cup grated Parmesan cheese

1 teaspoon salt

1 teaspoon dried thyme

1 teaspoon dried basil

¼ cup olive oil

## Directions

1. Preheat the oven to 400 degrees F. Cut the chicken into 1½-inch cubes. Set aside.

2. In a bowl, mix together the popped kiwicha, cheese, salt, thyme, and basil. Dip the chicken pieces into olive oil to coat, and roll each in the kiwicha mixture to evenly bread the chicken.

3. Place the coated chicken pieces on a lightly greased cookie sheet and bake for 20 minutes, turning the chicken over after 10 minutes.

**Per Serving:** Kcal 191, Protein 16g, Carb 5g, Fat 12g, Sodium 766mg, Dietary Fiber 1g
**Daily Values:** Fiber 2%, Vit C 0%, Vit A 1%, Vit D 0%, Calcium 8%, Iron 3%

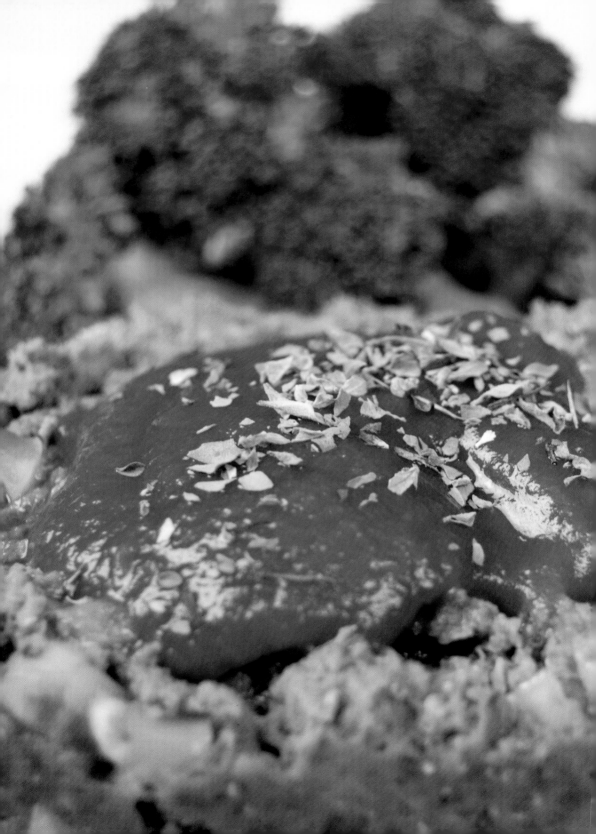

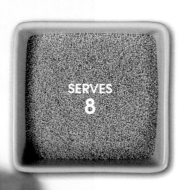

# KIWICHA MEAT LOAF

*Most meat loaf recipes call for some sort of bread or panko to fill out and fluff up the beef blend. Here, we just substituted popped kiwicha for a light and satisfying take on the comfort classic.*

**SERVES 8**

## Ingredients

¾ cup chopped onion
¾ cup chopped celery
2 pounds extra lean ground beef (4% fat)
1½ cups popped kiwicha (3¼ tablespoons raw kiwicha)
½ cup egg whites
¼ cup milk
⅛ cup ketchup
2 tablespoons dried oregano
2 teaspoons salt
2 teaspoons pepper

## Directions

1. Preheat the oven to 350 degrees F. Mix all of the ingredients in a bowl and add salt and pepper to taste. Transfer the mixture to a meat-loaf dish, or shape it into a log on a baking sheet. Bake for 60 minutes. Slice and serve.

*gluten-free*

**Per Serving:** Kcal 196, Protein 27g, Carb 6g, Fat 6g, Sodium 154mg, Dietary Fiber 1g
**Daily Values:** Fiber 4%, Vit C 4%, Vit A 2%, Vit D 1%, Calcium 4%, Iron 18%

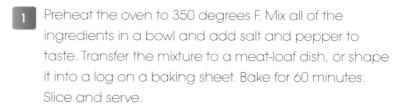

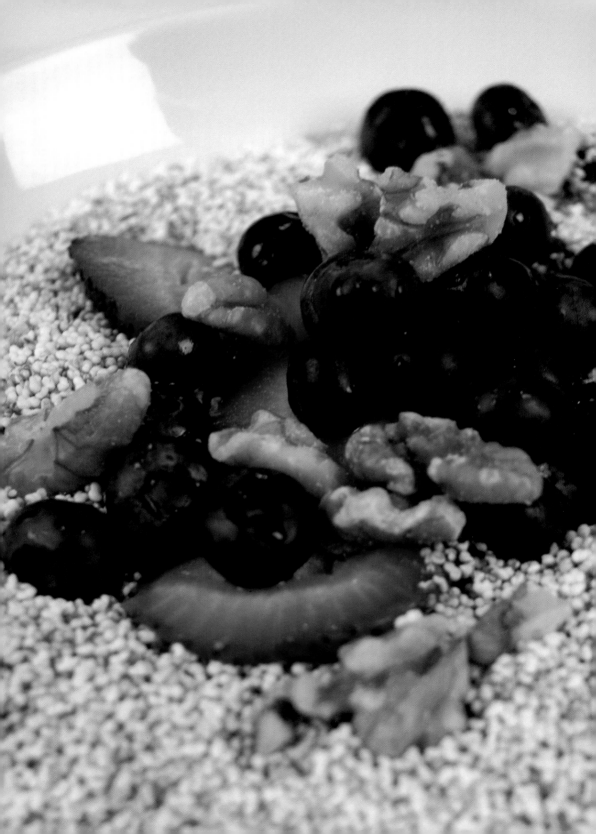

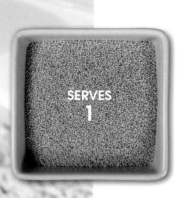

**SERVES
1**

# POPPED KIWICHA BREAKFAST CEREAL

*Sounds simple, and it is. Just use your popped kiwicha in place of your favorite cereal, and add berries or bananas to sweeten.*

## Ingredients

1 cup popped kiwicha (3 tablespoons raw)
1 cup milk of choice
1 cup berries of choice, or 1 banana, sliced

## Directions

**1** Add the milk and berries or bananas to the kiwicha and enjoy!

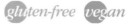 *gluten-free* *vegan*

**Per Serving:** Kcal 137, Protein 5g, Carb 24g, Fat 2g, Sodium 8mg, Dietary Fiber 3g
**Daily Values:** Fiber 14%, Vit C 3%, Vit A 0%, Vit D 0%, Calcium 6%, Iron 15%

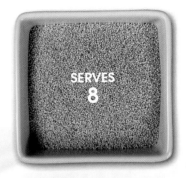

**SERVES 8**

# KIWICHA GRANOLA BARS WITH LUCUMA AND PICHUBERRIES

*Once you learn how to make these tasty, textured granola bars, there's no need to go for store-bought ever again. We paired kiwicha with pichuberries and lucuma for a triple boost of power foods, but you can also add or substitute your favorite fruits, nuts, and grains to this base recipe.*

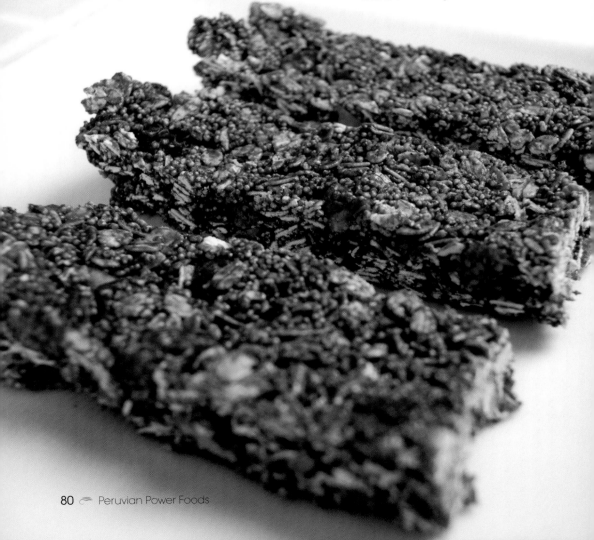

## Ingredients

1½ cups old-fashioned oats
2 cups popped kiwicha (about 6
   tablespoons raw kiwicha)
½ cup chopped walnuts
½ cup dried pichuberries
½ cup lucuma

½ cup brown rice syrup
1 teaspoon vanilla extract
1 teaspoon sea salt
½ to 1 teaspoon cinnamon
1 tablespoon cocoa powder

## Directions

1. Preheat the oven to 325 degrees F and place the oven rack in the middle of the oven. Line a baking pan with parchment paper, leaving excess paper over the sides. Lightly coat the paper with nonstick cooking spray or butter.

2. In a large bowl, mix the oats, popped kiwicha, nuts, dried fruit, and lucuma together.

3. In a small saucepan, warm the rice syrup over medium heat until it is just loose and ready to pour. Mix in the vanilla extract, salt, cinnamon, and cocoa powder. Pour the syrup mixture over the dry ingredients, and thoroughly mix with a spatula.

4. Pour the mixture into the prepared pan, and firmly press the mixture in the pan. For chewy granola bars, bake for 20 to 25 minutes. For a crunchy granola bar, bake for 25 to 30 minutes. As soon as you remove the pan from the oven, press the baked mixture down again with a lightly oiled spatula. Allow to cool completely in the pan.

5. With a very sharp knife cut the cooled bars into eight even servings. Store them in an airtight container, in the refrigerator, for 5 to 7 days.

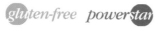 

*gluten-free* **powerstar** *vegan*

**Per Serving:** Kcal 324, Protein 10g, Carb 55g, Fat 7g, Sodium 306mg, Dietary Fiber 6g
**Daily Values:** Fiber 25%, Vit C 1%, Vit A 0%, Vit D 0%, Calcium 4%, Iron 13%

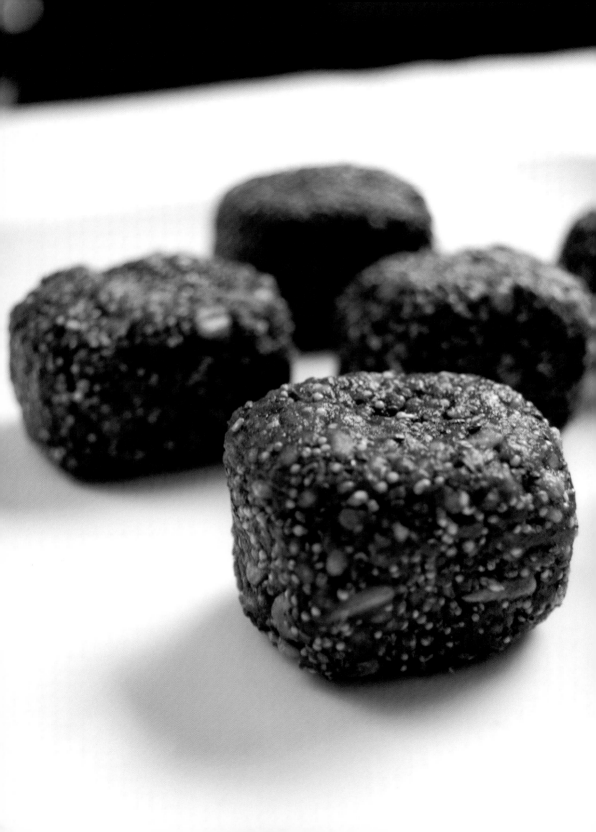

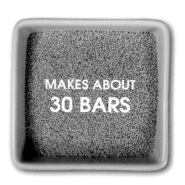

# NO-BAKE KIWICHA BARS

**MAKES ABOUT 30 BARS**

*What's better than a bar you don't have to bake? It's easy to assemble this tasty combination of power foods for a grab-and-go energy booster, a breakfast bar, or even a healthy dessert.*

## Ingredients

2 cups popped kiwicha (6 tablespoons raw kiwicha)

2 cups cooked quinoa

½ cup chia seeds

½ cup sunflower seeds

1 teaspoon kosher salt

1 cup sunflower seed butter

½ cup yacon

2 ounces pureed dates (using food processor, puree 3 to 4 pitted dates)

½ cup maca

## Directions

**1** Combine all of the dry ingredients in a bowl. Stir in the sunflower seed butter, yacon, dates, and maca until well combined.

**2** Press the mixture into an 8 x 8 inch pan and refrigerate until firm. Cut into 2-inch squares and enjoy! Store in an airtight container, in the refrigerator, for 5 to 7 days.

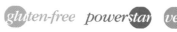 

**Per Serving:** Kcal 126, Protein 4g, Carb 15g, Fat 7g, Sodium 79mg, Dietary Fiber 3g
**Daily Values:** Fiber 10%, Vit C 2%, Vit A 0%, Vit D 0%, Calcium 5%, Iron 8%

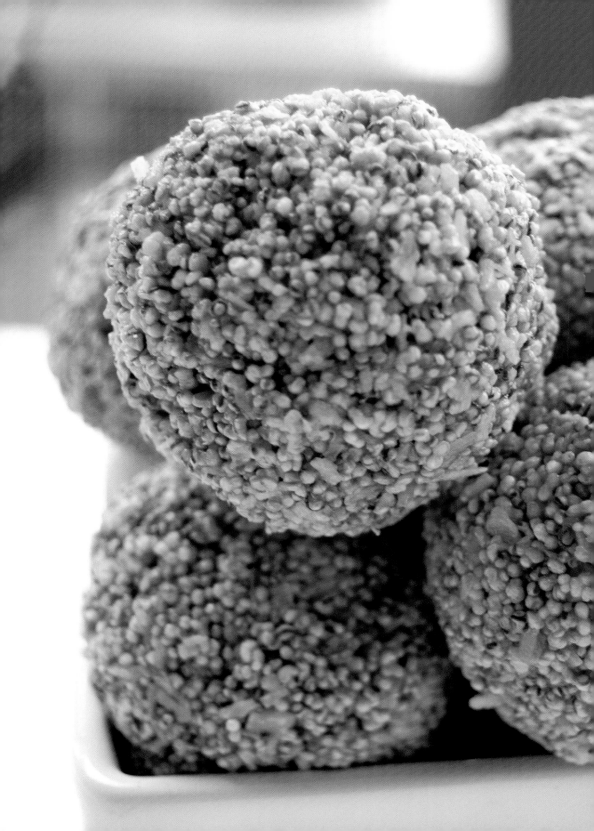

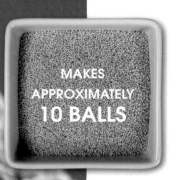

**MAKES APPROXIMATELY 10 BALLS**

# DULCE DE LECHE KIWICHA CRISPIES

*Consider this our less-processed take on the classic American Rice Krispie treat. These kiwicha treats bring some Peruvian flair with the rich flavor of dulce de leche and a kiss of coconut flakes.*

## Ingredients

2½ cups popped kiwicha (6¼ tablespoons raw kiwicha)
½ cup dulce de leche
¼ cup honey
½ cup shredded unsweetened coconut

## Directions

**1** In a large bowl, combine all of the ingredients and thoroughly mix with your hands. Once the mixture is evenly incorporated, transfer it to an 8 x 8 inch baking dish and press down with a spatula to pack the mixture tightly.

**2** Refrigerate for 1 to 2 hours, or until the mixture has hardened slightly.

**3** With your hands, form 2-inch balls. Store the kiwicha krispies in an airtight container, in the refrigerator, for 5 to 7 days.

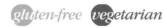

*gluten-free* *vegetarian*

**Per Serving:** Kcal 158, Protein 3g, Carb 22g, Fat 7g, Sodium 5mg, Dietary Fiber 2g
**Daily Values:** Fiber 8%, Vit C 1%, Vit A 0%, Vit D 0%, Calcium 1%, Iron 5%

# 5 ⌒ AVOCADO

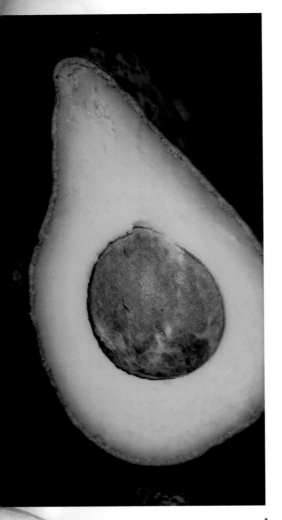

## OVERVIEW

**AVOCADOS ARE VERY FAMILIAR** to us in the United States. In fact, today we are the third-largest producer of the crop behind Mexico and Brazil. As most of us in the United States know, the avocado is a fruit that is the size of a small mango. Its bumpy black skin encases pale green "meat" that, once ripe, achieves one of the smoothest, most satisfying textures of all natural ingredients.

Many people identify avocado flesh as "good fat," which indeed it is. Avocados are packed with almost 20 essential nutrients, including fiber, vitamins B and E, folic acid, and potassium. Avocados

Although the avocado is originally from Central America, the Incas discovered it in Ecuador—specifically in the province of Palta—and brought it down the Pacific Coast to their homeland. To this day, avocados are still known as "Palta" in Peru.

also promote optimal nutrition by helping the body absorb more fat-soluble substances, like lutein, as well as alpha- and beta-carotene. Avocados have anticancer benefits, and they fight inflammation, which can cause a host of different diseases.

*The most common use of avocados may be in guacamole, the popular creation from the Aztecs in Mexico, but an avocado is wonderful sliced on its own, on top of eggs, chili, soup, salads, sandwiches—you name it. Recently, health advocates have also discovered many innovative ways to use avocados as a thickening agent in smoothies and creamy desserts like mousses and pies, where it replaces dairy ingredients for vegans and lactose-intolerant eaters.*

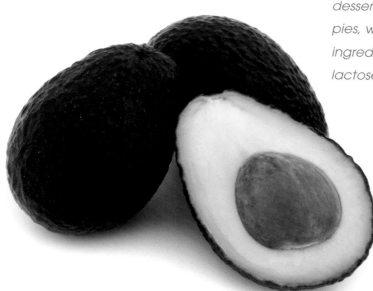

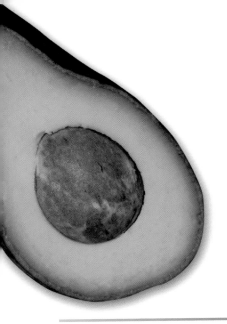

# NUTRITION & HEALTH
## BENEFITS

Avocados are rich in essential nutrients, including fiber, folic acid, potassium, and vitamins B and E. They are high in antioxidants, carotenoids, lutein, and tocopherols. They are also low in cholesterol and low in sodium.

Many studies show that a diet rich in avocados and its many phytochemicals may help to prevent cancer. Avocados fight the bacteria that cause stomach cancer, they have been proven to kill oral cancer cells, and they inhibit prostate cancer cells from growing and spreading.

Avocados contain the phytochemicals carotenoid and lutein, which act as anti-inflammatory agents.

Eating avocados can help decrease blood triglycerides and increase HDL (the "good" cholesterol). Both short- and long-term studies show that eating avocados also decreases high blood pressure, which lowers the risk of developing cardiovascular disease.

Avocados help control type 2 diabetes by reducing blood glucose values and long-term high blood sugar indicators.

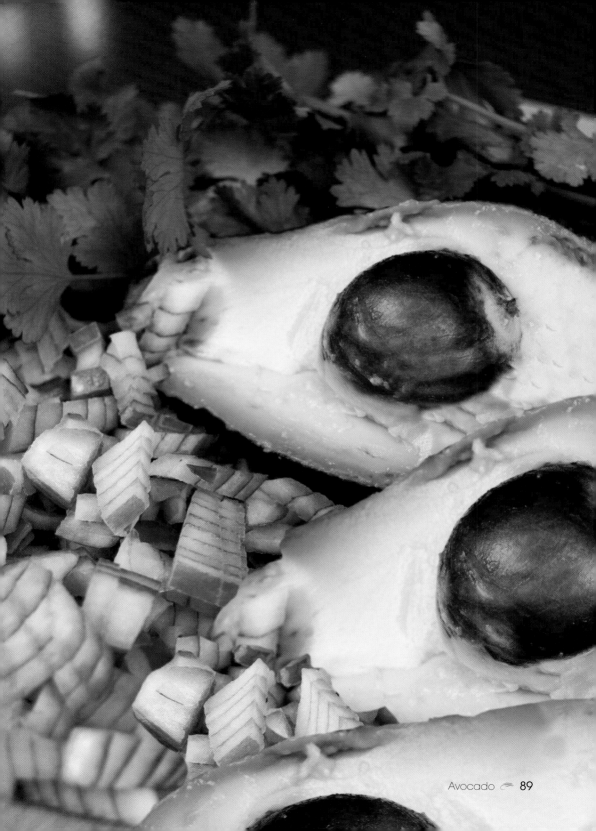

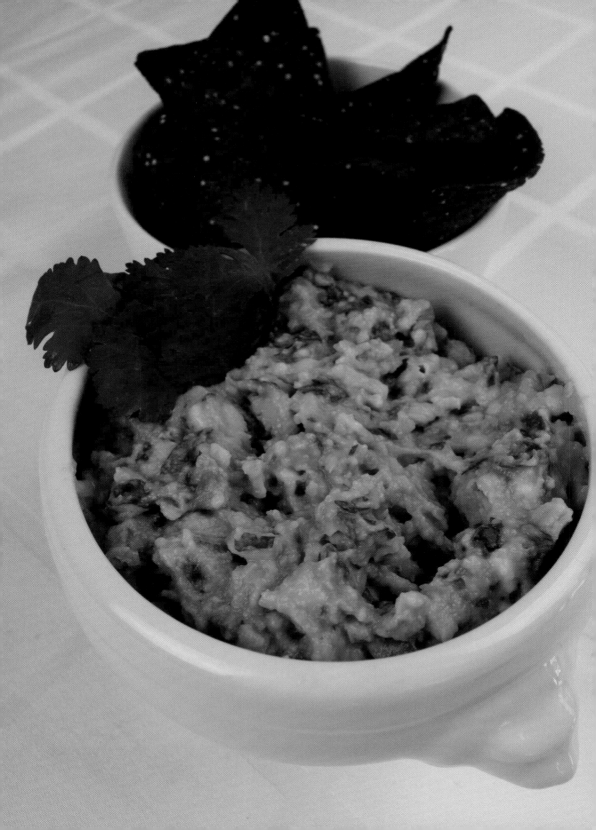

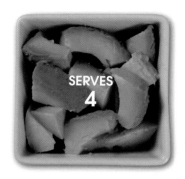

# AMAZONIAN GUAC

*After visiting the river port of Iquitos in the Amazon, we returned to Lima and sought out the world's first high-end restaurant serving Amazonian cuisine, Amaz. There we noticed the chefs were using avocados plentifully, so we decided to create an Amazonian version of classic Mexican guacamole. We added sacha inchi oil to bolster the antioxidant power of this delicious dish and to include essential omega-3s. It's the same flavor you love with a little hint of grassy sweetness.*

## Ingredients

3 medium avocados
Juice of 3 limes
2 tablespoons sacha inchi oil
¼ cup finely diced shallots
¼ cup chopped cilantro plus an extra sprig for garnish
Salt to taste

## Directions

1. Slice the avocados in half lengthwise, remove the pits, and peel off the skin.

2. In a medium-sized bowl, mash the avocado flesh with a fork. Add the lime juice, sacha inchi oil, shallots, cilantro, and salt. Garnish with a cilantro sprig and serve with blue corn chips for even more nutritional power.

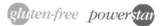 *gluten-free* **powerstar** *vegan*

**Per Serving:** Kcal 246, Protein 2g, Carb 12g, Fat 22g, Sodium 155mg, Dietary Fiber 7g
**Daily Values:** Fiber 28%, Vit C 28%, Vit A 7%, Vit D 0%, Calcium 2%, Iron 4%

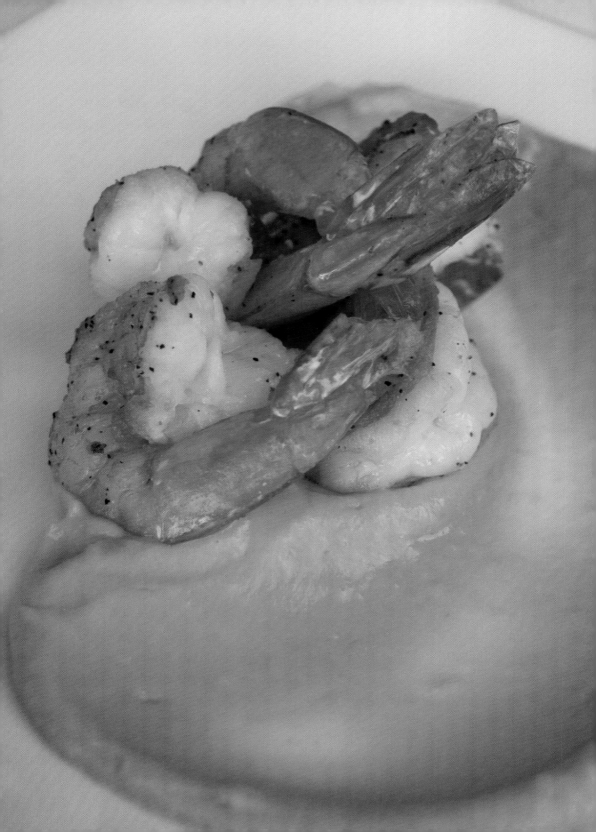

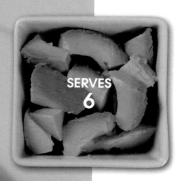

**SERVES 6**

# AVOCADO MOUSSE

*Waterbar is an elegant seafood restaurant on San Francisco's bayside Embarcadero waterfront. We asked Chef Jason D'Angelo how he likes to combine avocados with seafood dishes, and he shared this simple but versatile mousse. While it pairs beautifully with prawns and all kinds of white fish, you can also spread it on the plate as a design element for presentation.*

## Ingredients

2 avocados
2 limes
½ cup buttermilk
Salt to taste

## Directions

1. Slice the avocados in half lengthwise, remove the pits, and peel off the skin. Juice 2 limes.

2. Combine the avocado, lime juice, and buttermilk in a blender, and thoroughly mix until you have a whipped mousse that should be light in texture and weight. You can also place the ingredients in a bowl and use a hand mixer instead of the blender. Season with salt.

**Per Serving:** Kcal 89, Protein 2g, Carb 7g, Fat 7g, Sodium 122mg, Dietary Fiber 4g
**Daily Values:** Fiber 15%, Vit C 18%, Vit A 2%, Vit D 0%, Calcium 4%, Iron 2%

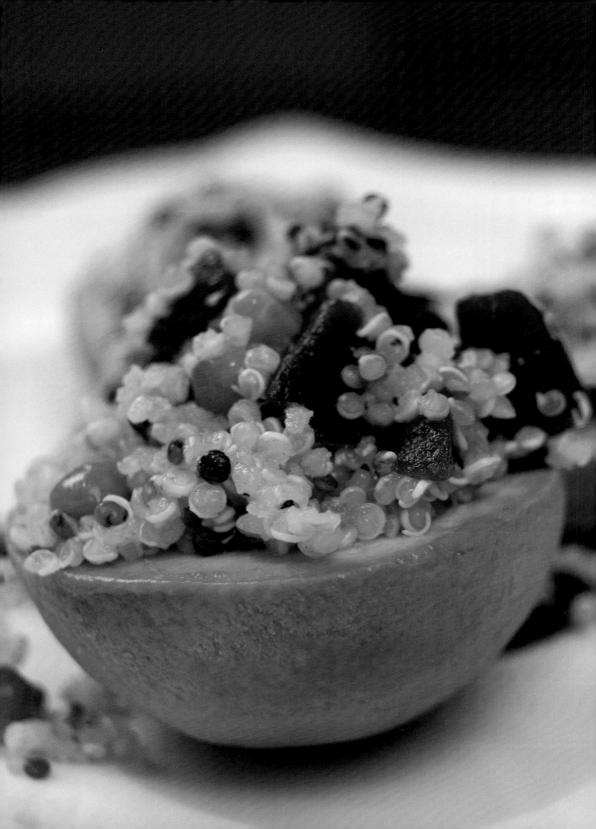

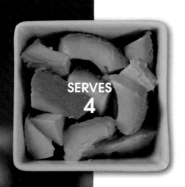

SERVES
4

# PERUVIAN STUFFED AVOCADO

*Stuffing avocados is a great way to create a well-balanced entrée. In this recipe, we used quinoa for protein content, peas and beets for smart carbs, and lime juice for tangy flavor. It's easy, colorful, and superhealthy to boot.*

## Ingredients

2 avocados
½ cup cooked quinoa
¼ cup peas, fresh or frozen
¼ cup diced steamed beets
1 tablespoon lime juice
Salt and pepper to taste

## Directions

1. Slice the avocados in half lengthwise, remove the pits, and peel off the skin. Set the avocado halves aside.

2. Combine the quinoa, peas, beets, and lime juice in a bowl and gently fold together until thoroughly mixed. Season with salt and pepper.

3. Fill the avocados with the quinoa mixture and serve.

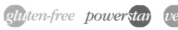 *gluten-free* **powerstar** *vegan*

Per Serving: Kcal 152, Protein 3g, Carb 13g, Fat 11g, Sodium 14mg, Dietary Fiber 6g
Daily Values: Fiber 24%, Vit C 15%, Vit A 4%, Vit D 0%, Calcium 2%, Iron 6%

AVOCADO RECIPES

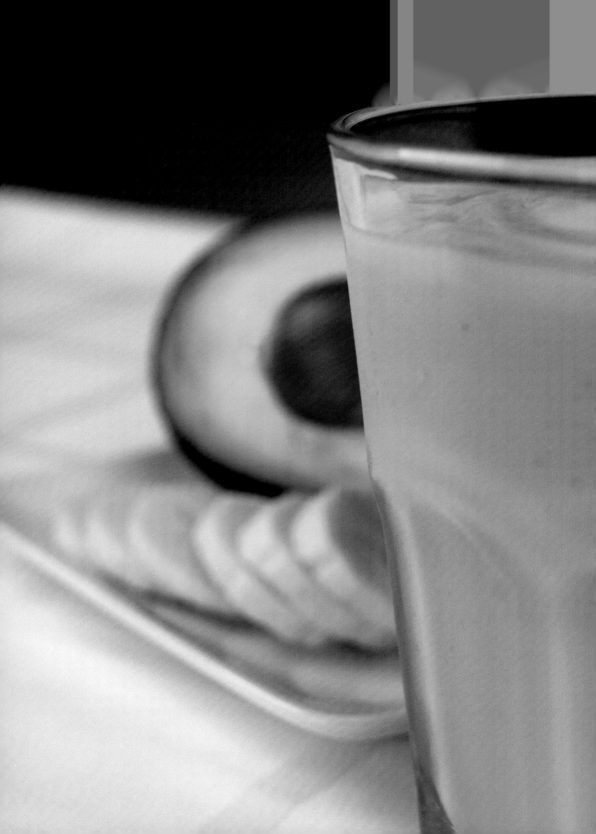

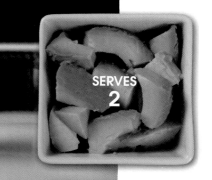

**SERVES 2**

# AVOCADO SMOOTHIE

*Besides being delicious on its own or as a featured element of a dish, avocado makes a great behind-the-scenes thickening agent. Add it to a smoothie and you'll notice a thick, luscious texture that also imparts great health benefits. The flavor here is all banana and orange, but the avocado creates next-level creaminess.*

## Ingredients

½ avocado
½ banana
¼ cup nonfat plain Greek yogurt
1 cup fresh orange juice
2 tablespoons honey
½ to 1 cup ice

## Directions

 Combine all of the ingredients in a blender and mix until smooth.

 gluten-free 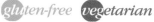 vegetarian

**Per Serving:** Kcal 217, Protein 4g, Carb 41g, Fat 5g, Sodium 19mg, Dietary Fiber 3g
**Daily Values:** Fiber 13%, Vit C 113%, Vit A 6%, Vit D 0%, Calcium 2%, Iron 3%

# 6 ⌐ AJI

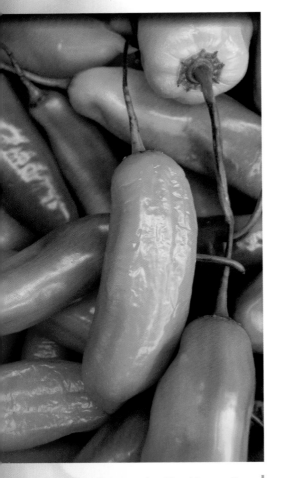

## OVERVIEW

**ALSO KNOWN AS THE** *aji amarillo* or the "yellow chili pepper" of Peru's Andes mountains, this popular pepper has been a staple of the Peruvian diet since the days of the Incas. Today it is still the most popular pepper in Peruvian cuisine.

The aji has a fruity, subtle, smoky flavor and a medium heat level. It grows to 4 to 5 inches in length and matures to a bright orange. It carries some spiciness, but doesn't impart a burning sensation. These days it is widely available in powdered form, commonly found in Latin markets or online.

Aji is the most critical ingredient in Peruvian cooking. While the French begin many recipes with a *mirepoix* mix of onion, celery, and carrot, Peruvians begin with *aderezo*, which is aji peppers, onion, garlic, and oil. Most Peruvian soups, stews, and sautés begin with this classic mixture.

Besides delivering superlative flavor, this pepper packs high levels of capsaicin, a natural compound that has been shown to help people burn more calories with regular consumption. The aji pepper has also been shown to fight cancer cells, particularly those associated with prostate cancer.

*All across South America, peppers are a common ingredient in the local cuisine. The aji stands out as being exceptionally versatile, since its characteristics are more fruity and smoky than spicy. It's great in sauces as well as incorporated with sautéed and grilled dishes.*

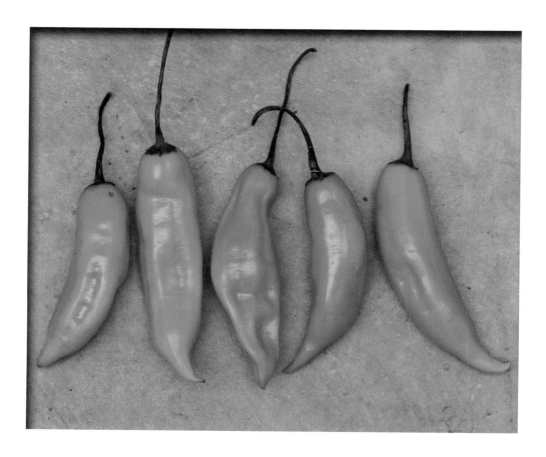

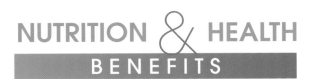

# NUTRITION & HEALTH
## BENEFITS

### ANTICANCER

### SUPPORTS WEIGHT LOSS

Aji peppers are rich in vitamins A, B, and C. The active ingredient is capsaicin, which delivers many of the myriad health benefits.

Capsaicin helps with weight management. While the exact reasons remain unclear, research reveals that capsaicin can increase energy, increase lipid oxidation, and reduce appetite. Studies show people who eat chilies containing capsaicin burn calories for up to 15 minutes longer because of all the heat produced in the body. In fact, studies show that when eaten regularly, capsaicin can effect marked weight loss over a one- to two-year period.

Studies show capsaicin prevents cancer cells from multiplying.

Capsaicin has been proven to slow the growth of prostate cancer cells.

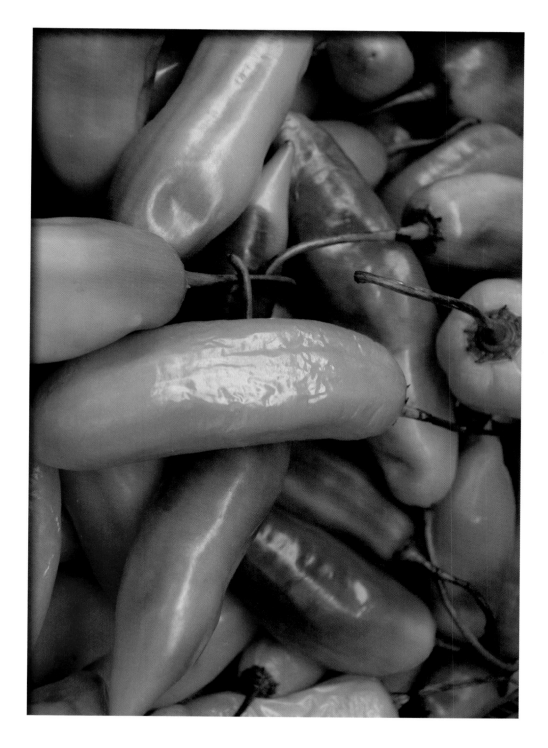

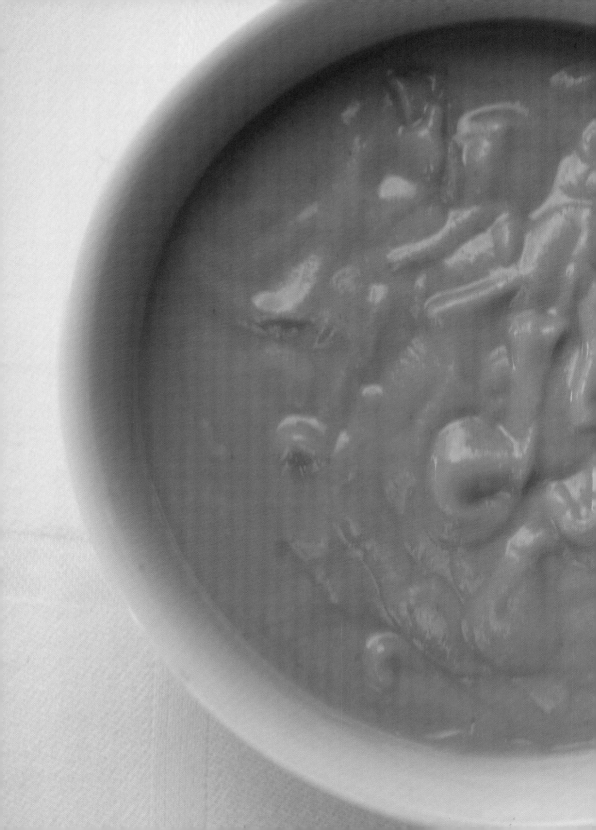

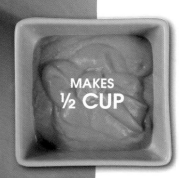

**MAKES ½ CUP**

# AJI SAUCE

*These days, aji sauce is available in most Latino stores or online, but if you find ajis in a local market—either fresh or frozen—this is a simple recipe to make your own fresh sauce.*

## Ingredients

8 aji chili peppers
1 tablespoon olive oil
3 tablespoons water
Salt to taste

## Directions

1. Cut the peppers in half and pull the seeds and core from the center. Place the peppers in a small pot with water and boil for 10 minutes.

2. Strain the chili mixture and pulse it in the blender with the oil and the water until you achieve a smooth consistency.

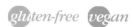

*gluten-free* *vegan*

**AJI RECIPES**

**Per Serving:** Kcal 20, Protein 0g, Carb 1g, Fat 1g, Sodium 34mg, Dietary Fiber 0g
**Daily Values:** Fiber 0%, Vit C 0%, Vit A 0%, Vit D 0%, Calcium 0%, Iron 0%

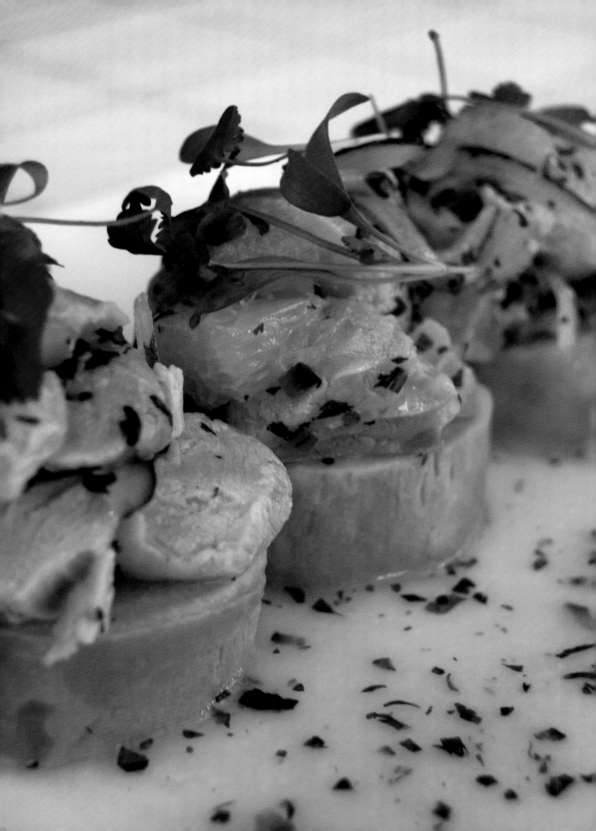

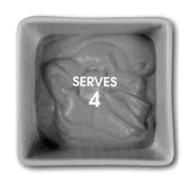

# SEASIDE CEVICHE

*The most important aspect of ceviche is, of course, that it's as fresh as can be. And that is always dependent on getting the best catch available. Once you've secured a beautiful piece of fish, this is our chef-certified perfect preparation from Jason D'Angelo of Waterbar in San Francisco.*

## Ingredients

3 to 4 sweet potatoes, halved

4 ounces raw fish (we recommend sole, sea bass, or thinly sliced halibut)

Juice of 2 oranges

Juice of 2 limes

1 teaspoon aji paste

2 tablespoons diced orange segments

1½ teaspoons diced jalapeño

2 tablespoons finely diced red onion

1 tablespoon chopped cilantro

1 tablespoon extra virgin olive oil

Salt to taste

Microgreens to garnish (Any kind of small tender greens like arugula or watercress will do. You can find them in most expansive produce sections.)

## Directions

1  Boil the sweet potatoes over medium heat until thoroughly cooked (approximately 30 minutes until tender in the center). Set aside to cool.

2  Cut the fish into ½-inch squares. Place in a medium bowl. Add the orange juice, lime juice, and aji paste to the fish and lightly stir. Add the orange segments, jalapeño, red onion, cilantro, and the oil, and lightly combine. Season with salt.

3  Slice the cooled sweet potato into 1- to 2-inch-thick slices, arrange on a plate, and place the ceviche over them. Garnish with microgreens.

*gluten-free*

**AJI RECIPES**

**Per Serving:** Kcal 184, Protein 7g, Carb 30g, Fat 4g, Sodium 86mg, Dietary Fiber 4g
**Daily Values:** Fiber 15%, Vit C 53%, Vit A 326%, Vit D 0%, Calcium 5%, Iron 5%

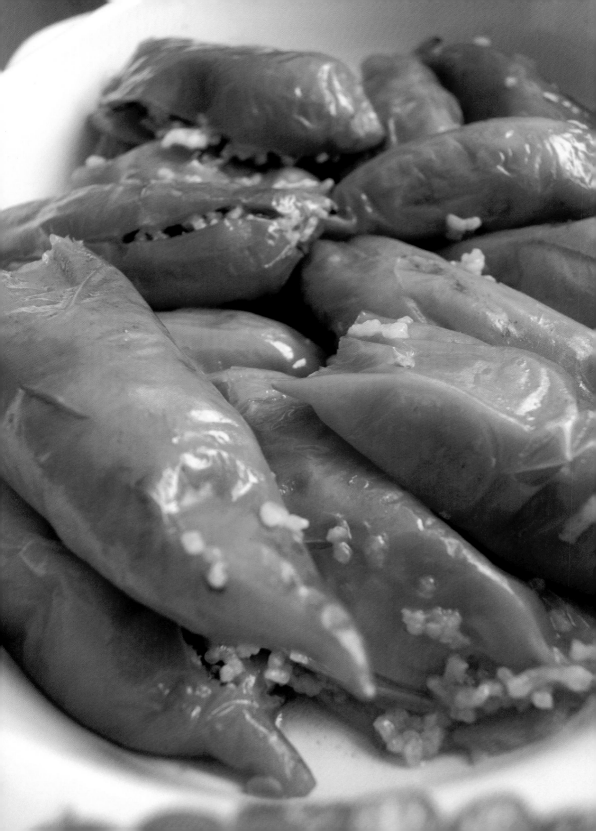

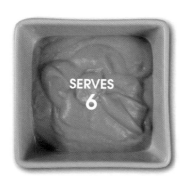

SERVES
6

# AJI RELLENO

*Almost every culture around the world has some version of a stuffed pepper. Here, we share a standard Peruvian take, pairing the always popular aji with a little cumin for more depth and interest.*

## Ingredients

6 medium to large aji chili
    peppers
½ cup dry rice
1 cup raw ground meat
½ cup chopped parsley

1 teaspoon cumin
2 garlic cloves, chopped
2 tablespoons tomato paste
3 cups chicken broth
Salt and pepper to taste

## Directions

1. Prepare and clean the aji peppers: Cut off the tops, open them using your hands and the stub of a knife; remove all the seeds and wash the peppers well.

2. Thoroughly mix together the rice, meat, parsley, cumin, garlic, tomato paste, and salt and pepper. Fill the peppers halfway with the rice mixture, and place them in a pot. Pour 1 cup of the chicken broth over the peppers. Cook, covered, for 25 to 30 minutes. Toward the end of the 25-minute cooking time, check to see if the rice is cooked inside of the aji. If it needs more time, continue adding more broth, ½ cup at a time, until the rice is cooked.

AJI RECIPES

gluten-free

**Per Serving:** Kcal 139, Protein 11g, Carb 15g, Fat 2g, Sodium 399mg, Dietary Fiber 1g
**Daily Values:** Fiber 2%, Vit C 15%, Vit A 10%, Vit D 0%, Calcium 3%, Iron 13%

# 7 ⌒ CAMU CAMU

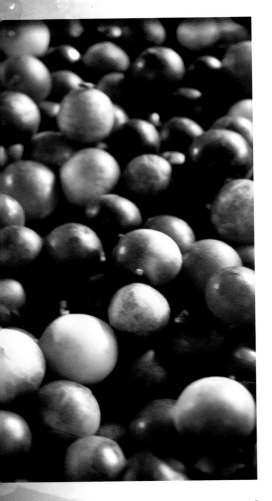

Native Amazonian people have understood the benefits of camu camu for centuries. In addition to relying on it as a food source, they use it to relieve pain, treat infection, and keep their hair shiny. They also believe in camu camu's power to promote a long life.

## OVERVIEW

**CAMU CAMU IS A TROPICAL FRUIT** that varies between the size of a large grape and a small nectarine. Commonly found in the Amazonian jungle, this prized resource is used in a vast array of food preparations when it comes in season from November to May. It's usually harvested by canoe in the rainforest, as it grows during the rainy season when waters are high or flooding.

The camu berry is one of the world's most potent sources of vitamin C—packing more than 60 times the amount per serving than the almighty orange. Just think, oranges often have around 1,000 ppm (parts per million) of vitamin C, while the camu berry can have concentrations as high as 50,000 ppm or about 2 grams of vitamin C per 100 grams of fruit. Translation: the camu berry can offer 50 times more vitamin C than an orange on an ounce-for-ounce basis. Camu also provides ten times more iron, three times more niacin, twice as much riboflavin, and 50 percent more phosphorus than its citrus competitors.

Vitamin C is known to help with immunity, tissue repair, and healing, as well as with cancer and cataract prevention. And because the vitamin is naturally occurring in camu camu, the body better absorbs the nutrient than it does from a tablet of the same concentration. Camu camu appears to be more effective in delivering ascorbic acid than synthetic vitamin C, and also contains bioflavenoids and other phytochemicals.

Vitamin C is complex; it's not just a single, isolated chemical in its natural form. It is delivered through power foods like camu in combination with several different supporting phytochemicals that make the positive effect of vitamin C even more powerful than when taken alone. High-density foods like camu give us the highest nutritional value possible through single sources.

Camu powder made from pulp is a convenient form that is often available in health food stores.

*Camu camu has a slightly sour taste, but that doesn't stop Peruvian natives from using it in all kinds of dishes and drinks with a little added sweetener. Its flavor profile especially lends itself to jams, jellies, and sweets. It's also very popular in refreshing summer drinks and cocktails.*

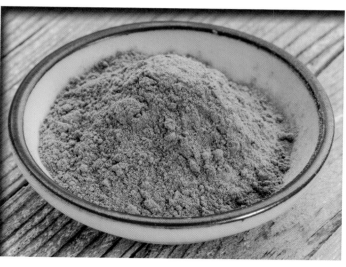

When we arrived in Iquitos—the heart of the Peruvian Amazon—camu camu was newly in season, and we found it everywhere, from ice cream to the pink frothy coolers garnished with tropical flowers at our hotel.

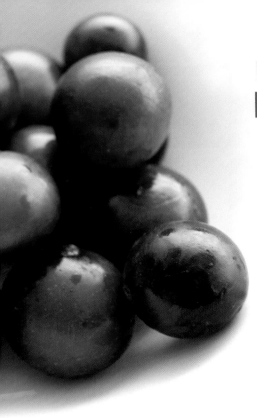

# NUTRITION & HEALTH

Camu camu contains a significant amount of vitamin C and is rich in beta-carotene, calcium, iron, niacin, phosphorus, potassium, riboflavin, and thiamin. It's also loaded with antioxidants, such as anthocyanins, and it has a higher content of essential amino acids than other fruits.

Vitamin C boosts immunity and supports collagen production, the main structural protein found in connective tissue. Vitamin C also helps to fight infection and supports healthy bones and teeth.

Vitamin C can help heal all kinds of wounds. From cuts and burns to broken bones and surgeries, vitamin C helps speed the healing process.

When it comes to cancer prevention, vitamin C delivers antioxidants that help protect cells from damage and mutation.

Vitamin C has been shown to fight coronary artery disease. It's a great source of anthocyanins, antioxidant pigments that fight inflammation, prevent cancer, improve vision, and help the brain stay healthy.

Vitamin C also helps prevent cataracts, a clouding of the lens of the eye that can cause blindness in older people.

Camu camu can also help protect your brain from neurodegenerative disorders. Many such diseases are caused by oxidative stress, so the high ascorbate levels in camu can guard against conditions such as Alzheimer's disease, dementia, Huntington's disease, ischemic stroke, and Parkinson's disease.

Because it is an anti-inflammatory agent, camu camu can be used to manage pain in disorders like rheumatoid arthritis.

If you're looking for anti-aging aids, meaning ingredients that help support skin elasticity and cellular maintenance, as well as brain function and vision, the camu berry is a winner on all fronts.

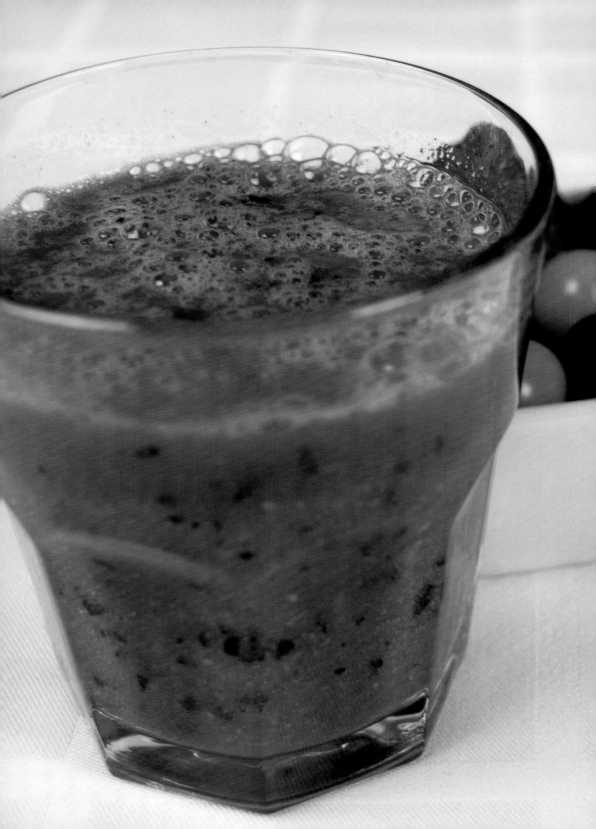

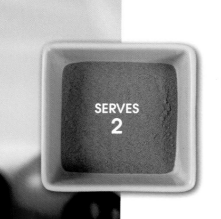

**SERVES
2**

# TRIPLE BERRY
# CAMU SHAKE

*This shake is a veritable vitamin powerhouse.
The combination of camu camu and pichuberries, not to mention all those other fruit favorites,
makes this a potent immunity booster and antioxidant injection.*

**CAMU CAMU RECIPES**

## Ingredients

1 cup pichuberries
1 cup blueberries
1 cup strawberries
2 teaspoons camu camu powder
16 ounces orange juice

## Directions

 Combine all of the ingredients in a blender and mix
until smooth.

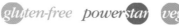 *gluten-free* **power*star*** *vegan*

**Per Serving:** Kcal 239, Protein 4g, Carb 55g, Fat 1g, Sodium 37mg, Dietary Fiber 4g
**Daily Values:** Fiber 17%, Vit C 1481%, Vit A 38%, Vit D 26%, Calcium 5%, Iron 16%

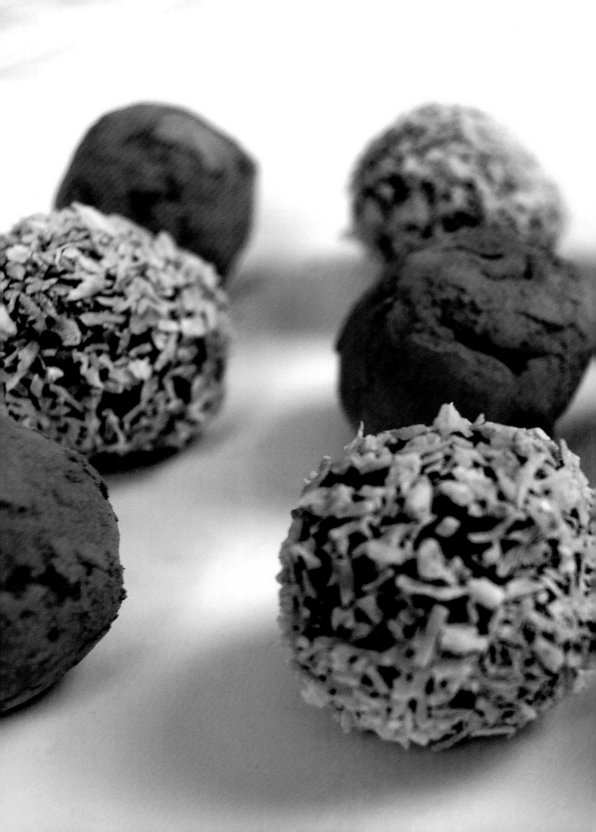

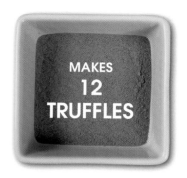

**MAKES**
**12**
**TRUFFLES**

# CAMU COCO TRUFFLE

*Easily our favorite sweet treat, these decadent truffles impart a deep, dark chocolate flavor, sweetened with antioxidant yacon syrup and kissed with tropical coconut flavor. This combination was inspired by Manuel's cousin, Natahli Giha, a well-known pastry chef in Lima.*

## Ingredients

3 ounces 70% or more dark chocolate

¼ cup coconut cream

1 tablespoon camu camu powder

2 tablespoons yacon syrup

3 ounces dried unsweetened coconut flakes

## Directions

1. Melt the dark chocolate in a double boiler.

2. In a separate saucepan, warm up the coconut cream with the camu camu and yacon. Heat until evenly combined, roughly 1 minute.

3. Combine the melted chocolate and the cream mixture until evenly incorporated. Refrigerate the mix until it becomes cool and hard, roughly 30 minutes.

4. Using your hands, form 1-inch truffle balls and roll them in coconut flakes. They can last up to one week in an airtight container in the refrigerator, but be sure to bring them to room temperature before serving.

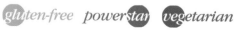

*gluten-free* *powerstar* *vegetarian*

**Per Serving:** Kcal 95, Protein 1g, Carb 9g, Fat 7g, Sodium 4mg, Dietary Fiber 1g
**Daily Values:** Fiber 5%, Vit C 295%, Vit A 0%, Vit D 0%, Calcium 0%, Iron 4%

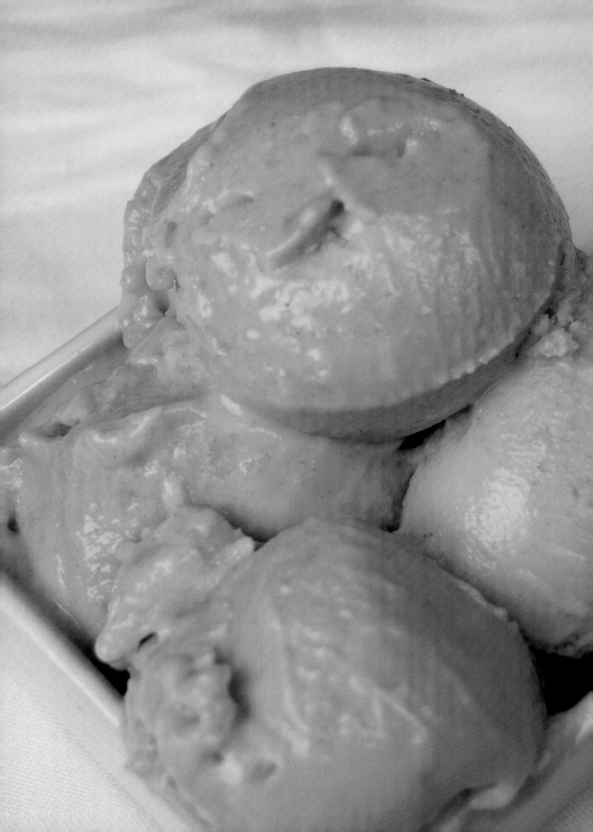

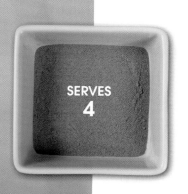

**SERVES 4**

# MANGO CAMU FROZEN YOGURT

*This is such a great way to enjoy the benefits of camu in a healthy, satisfying sweet. By using Greek yogurt as the base for this frozen dessert, you get all the enjoyment of eating homemade ice cream with none of the added fats or stabilizers.*

## Ingredients

2 cups chopped fresh mango
1 cup 2% plain Greek yogurt
¼ cup agave nectar
2 teaspoons camu camu powder

## Directions

1. Using a food processor or blender, puree the mangos. Add the remaining ingredients and blend until well mixed.

2. Cover and refrigerate the mixture for one to two hours. Then prepare according to your ice-cream maker's manufacturer instructions.

**NOTE:** *If you don't have an ice-cream maker, you can blend the refrigerated mix and use it for a smoothie, or put it into Popsicle molds.*

 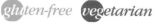
*gluten-free* *vegetarian*

Per Serving: Kcal 170, Protein 6g, Carb 34g, Fat 1g, Sodium 25mg, Dietary Fiber 1g
Daily Values: Fiber 6%, Vit C 628%, Vit A 14%, Vit D 0%, Calcium 7%, Iron 6%

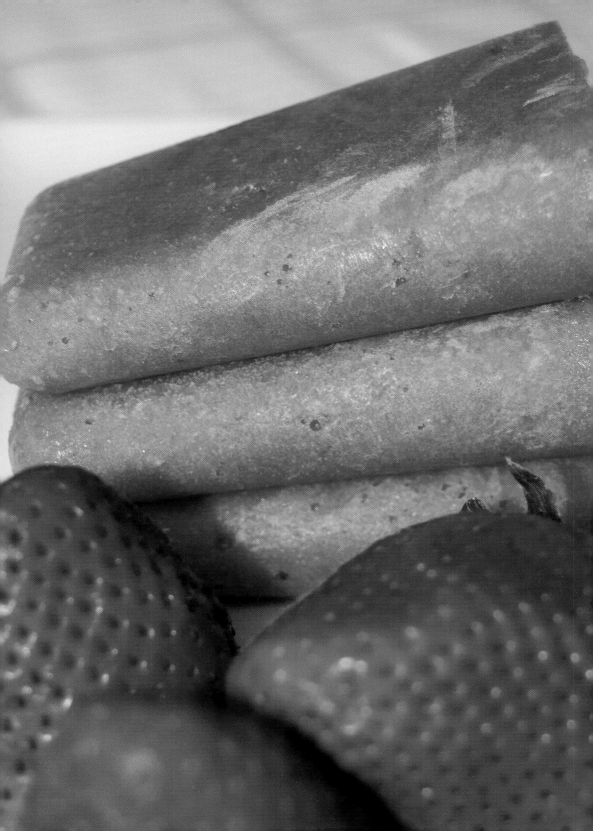

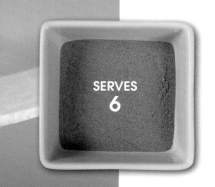

**SERVES
6**

# STRAWBERRY CAMU POPSICLES

*These frozen camu treats are as simple as they are delicious. Easy to assemble Popsicles make a refreshing, rewarding summer snack for kids and adults alike.*

## Ingredients

3 cups strawberries

5 tablespoons lime juice

½ cup agave

2 teaspoons camu camu powder

## Directions

**1** Combine all of the ingredients in a blender and mix until smooth. Transfer the mixture to Popsicle molds and freeze until firm, about 4 hours.

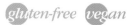 

Per Serving: Kcal 117, Protein 1g, Carb 29g, Fat 0g, Sodium 1mg, Dietary Fiber 1g
Daily Values: Fiber 6%, Vit C 470%, Vit A 1%, Vit D 0%, Calcium 1%, Iron 5%

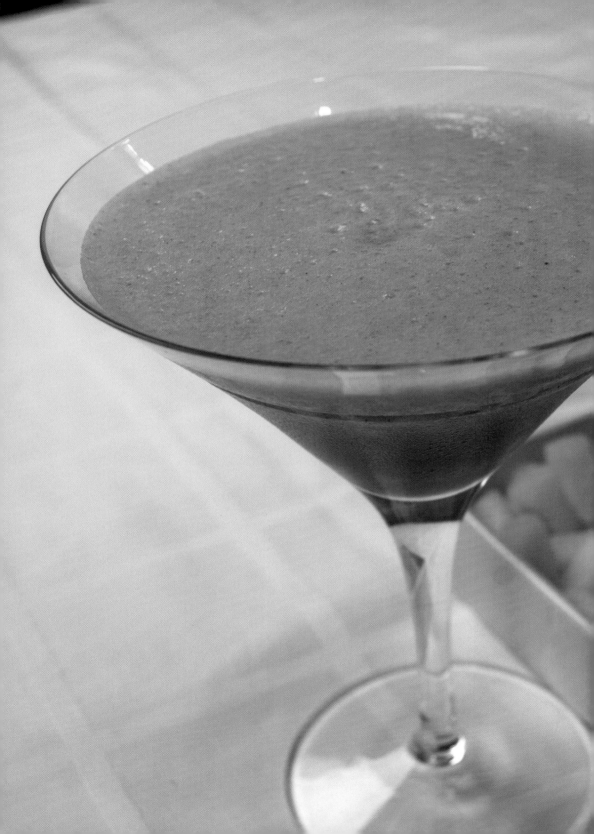

# CAMU PINEAPPLE PISCO

**SERVES 2**

*Camu is such a versatile and flavorful fruit, it just makes sense to build a tropical cocktail around it. Here, we've paired it with pisco, the official liquor of Peru, in a spirited summer sling.*

## Ingredients

1 cup frozen pineapple
1 tablespoon sugar or agave nectar
1 teaspoon camu camu powder
2 shots pisco
1 cup sparkling water

## Directions

1. Combine all of the ingredients in a blender and mix until smooth.

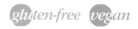
gluten-free vegan

Per Serving: Kcal 165, Protein 0g, Carb 23g, Fat 0g, Sodium 3mg, Dietary Fiber 1g
Daily Values: Fiber 4%, Vit C 652%, Vit A 2%, Vit D 0%, Calcium 2%, Iron 6%

# 8 ⌒ PURPLE CORN

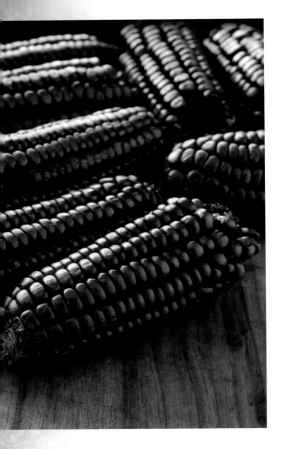

## OVERVIEW

**PURPLE CORN IS A** Peruvian power food cultivated in coastal areas, as well as in mountain highlands and valleys. It's one of over 3,000 corn varieties native to Peru—a staple of the native diet, dating back to the Incan civilization. As its name implies, it is purple in color—a deep vibrant hue derived from its nutrient-dense pigmentation. Purple foods owe their coloration to their high content of anthocyanin—a naturally occurring, water-soluble flavonoid that packs an antioxidant, antimicrobial, and anticarcinogenic punch. Purple corn is so laden with potent nutrients that it has an even higher anthocyanin content than fresh blueberries.

Mysteriously, perhaps magically, purple corn will lose its vibrant hue when planted in other countries, sometimes even presenting as yellow corn. Specialists surmise that the brilliant pigmentation development is attributed to something environmental in the soil, water, or climate of Peru, but the explanation is as yet unknown.

As with many of South America's abundant resources, purple corn almost became a lost crop, disregarded in favor of other grains and potatoes. But today, purple corn thrives in South America, as well as in American goods like "blue" corn chips, tortillas, and cornbread.

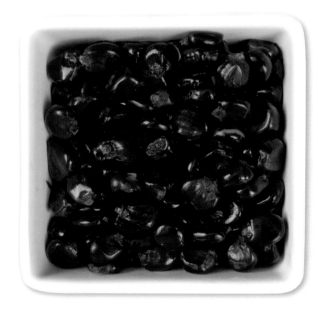

*For centuries, Peruvian people have soaked purple corn to make a brightly flavored sweet drink called chicha morada. It remains popular today and can be found everywhere from chic cevicherias and cocktail bars in Lima to small-town restaurants in the verdant Sacred Valley.*

*We used it as a base for drinks, sorbets, puddings, and Popsicles. Then we ground the cooked corn from the chicha drinks to make corn meal for bread and pancakes. Purple corn is as versatile and practical as it is tasty and nutritious. Of course, if you want to get the health benefits without pressing your own corn, you can find blue corn chips in most grocery stores today.*

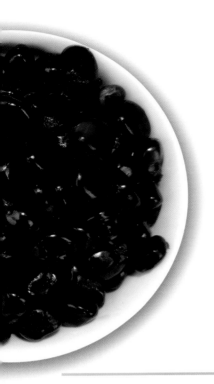

# NUTRITION & HEALTH
## BENEFITS

ANTICANCER

ANTI-INFLAMMATORY

BRAIN HEALTHY

HEART HEALTHY

IMPROVES VISION

PREVENTS LONG-TERM DIABETES DAMAGE

SUPPORTS IMMUNE SYSTEM

Purple corn is rich in phytonutrients, which protect the body from the impact of the environment, strengthen the body's immunity, and protect against carcinogens.

Purple corn can prevent long-term kidney damage in people with type 2 diabetes, by protecting renal cells. High blood sugar causes damage to the thin layers of cells surrounding the small blood vessels in the kidneys. This inflammation and fibrous tissue buildup contributes to end-stage kidney disease through kidney malfunction. Consuming purple corn has been shown to protect these thin layers of cells from getting this type of damage, thus helping to prevent long-term complications of type 2 diabetes.

Purple corn may also play a role in preventing prostate cancer as well as other cancers. One study performed at the University of Nagoya in Japan showed that purple corn pigment prevented the development of colon cancer.

Purple corn is a potent antioxidant, superior to many other common antioxidants. It may help protect many cells in the body, thus reducing damage to cells and reducing the risk of cancer cell formation.

The pigment has also been shown to decrease the inflammatory response of inflammation-causing diseases. It is also indicated to reduce blood pressure and blood cholesterol.

Anthocyanins have a potential to reduce the risk of heart disease, mostly likely due to decreased coagulation of platelets and increased circulation of HDL (good) cholesterol. Studies have also linked anthocyanins to vasodilation, or the widening of blood vessels.

Anthocyanins are also used in ophthalmology because they are known to help increase visual acuity and improve night vision.

Purple corn is a fabulous anti-aging agent as it also aids regeneration of connective tissue and the collagen formation required for healthy skin.

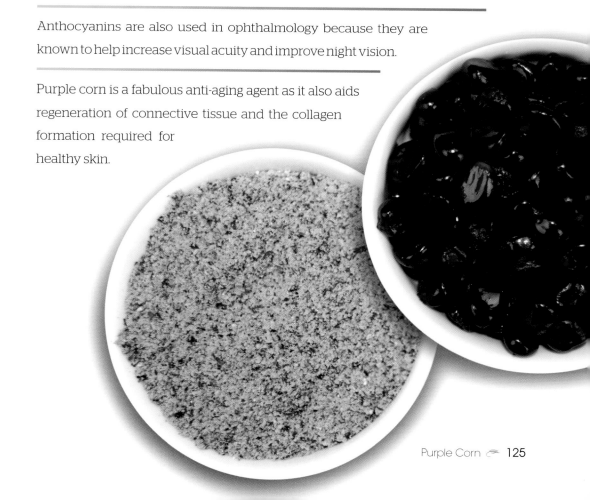

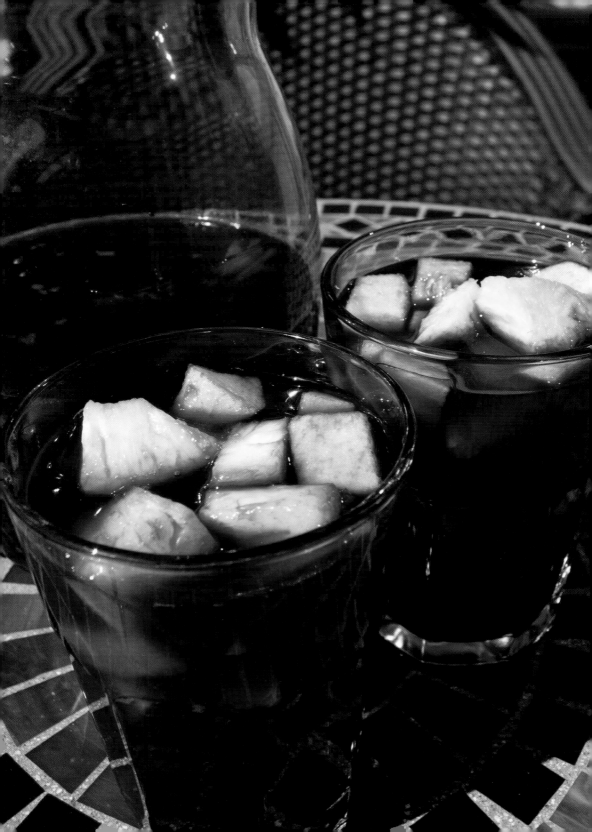

# CHICHA MORADA

**SERVES 12**

Chicha morada *is wildly popular in Peru, and most kids grow up drinking it as a cheaper, healthier alternative to soda. You'll find a version of it in almost every household. Do yourself a favor and try this classic Peruvian cooler. It's lightly spiced and clove scented, which brings a depth of flavor to the sweetness of the corn. Add a shot of pisco or some wine and it becomes a sophisticated sangria. Please note: this is not the same as Peruvian home-brewed beers called* chicha de jora.

## Ingredients

1 pound dried purple corn kernels
½ cup white sugar (you can add
   another ½ cup if you prefer it sweeter)
12 cups water
3 cinnamon sticks

½ cup lime juice
1 tablespoon whole cloves
1 green apple, peeled and diced
1 whole pineapple, diced
   (reserve the peel)

## Directions

1. In a large pot, add the purple corn, water, cinnamon sticks, cloves, and the pineapple peels. Heat over high heat until the mixture reaches a boil, then reduce the heat to medium-low and simmer for 45 minutes.

2. Remove the chicha from the heat and add the sugar and lime juice. Pour the mixture through a strainer into a large bowl, catching the remaining pulp. You can throw out the pulp or save it for use in other recipes like Purple Corn Lucuma Pancakes (see page 129) or Purple Corn Banana Bread (see page 131).

3. Refrigerate the mixture for about 3 hours or until cold. To serve, add ice, and the diced pineapple and apple to each glass.

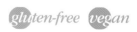 *gluten-free vegan*

**Per Serving:** Kcal 113, Protein 1g, Carb 27g, Fat 0g, Sodium 19mg, Dietary Fiber 2g
**Daily Values:** Fiber 8%, Vit C 23%, Vit A 1%, Vit D 0%, Calcium 2%, Iron 2%

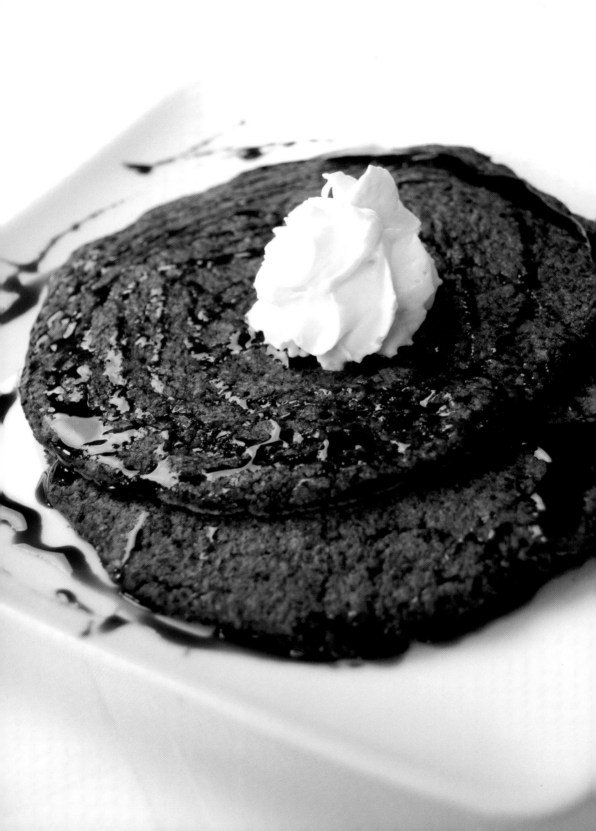

# PURPLE CORN LUCUMA PANCAKES

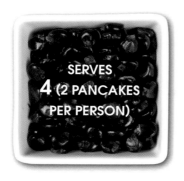

**SERVES 4** (2 PANCAKES PER PERSON)

*This is a wonderful combination of antioxidant ingredients that taste great together. Lucuma has a natural maplelike flavor, and corn makes a great textural base for waffles and pancakes. Replace your regular syrup with yacon (see page 238), and this dish becomes a power-packed breakfast.*

## Ingredients

2 cups corn meal—made from cooked purple corn kernels left over from *chicha morada* (1½ cups whole corn kernels make 2 cups corn meal)

½ teaspoon salt

2½ teaspoons baking powder

3 tablespoons lucuma

2 large eggs

½ cup milk

2 tablespoons applesauce

PURPLE CORN RECIPES

## Directions

1. Grind the purple corn in a coffee grinder until it forms a very small meal.

2. In a large bowl, sift together the purple corn meal, salt, baking powder, and lucuma.

3. In a separate bowl, whisk together the eggs, milk, and applesauce; add this to the flour mixture, stirring only until smooth.

4. On a hot, greased griddle, use about ¼ cup of batter for each pancake. Cook until bubbling, a little dry around the edges, and lightly browned on the bottom; turn and brown the other side. For extra nutrient power, serve with yacon syrup.

 *gluten-free* 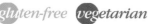 *vegetarian*

**Per Serving:** Kcal 119, Protein 6g, Carb 17g, Fat 3g, Sodium 349mg, Dietary Fiber 1g
**Daily Values:** Fiber 3%, Vit C 0%, Vit A 4%, Vit D 6%, Calcium 19%, Iron 6%

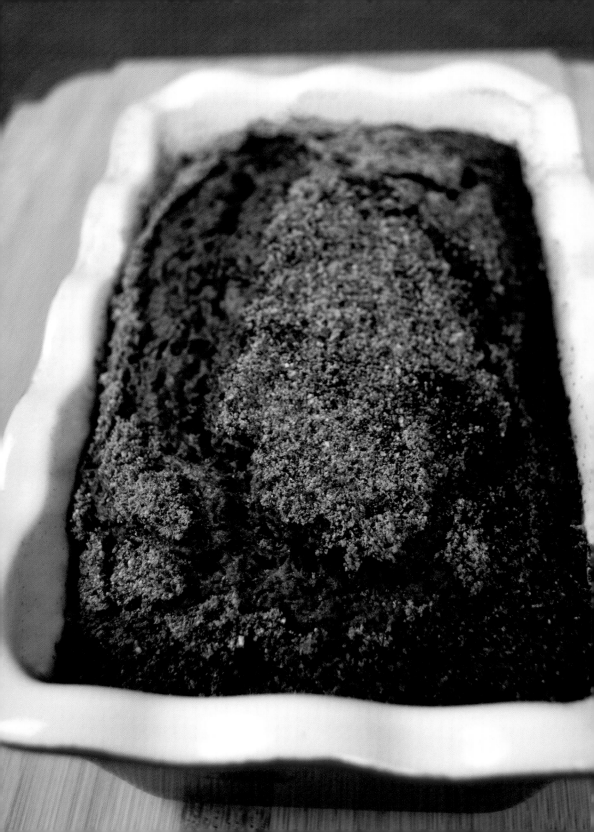

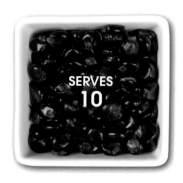

**SERVES 10**

# PURPLE CORN BANANA BREAD

*This enhanced banana bread is just bursting with the bright color and flavor of purple corn. Plus, it packs extra antioxidant benefits.*

## Ingredients

1 cup purple corn meal (made from cooked purple corn kernels leftover from chicha morada)

2 large bananas

½ cup agave nectar

½ cup applesauce

2 eggs

1 teaspoon vanilla extract

1 teaspoon baking soda

1 teaspoon baking powder

1 teaspoon salt

1 cup all-purpose flour

## Directions

1. Preheat the oven to 350 degrees F. Grind the purple corn in a coffee grinder until a very small grain meal is formed. Set aside.

2. Place the bananas in a large bowl and mash with an electric mixer. Stir in the agave nectar and let stand for 15 minutes. Add the applesauce and eggs and beat well. Add the vanilla, baking soda, baking powder, salt, and flour and mix thoroughly. Pour into a 9 x 5 inch loaf pan coated with nonstick vegetable spray and sprinkle the purple corn meal on top.

3. Bake about 60 minutes, or until a wooden toothpick inserted in the center of the loaf comes out clean. Remove from the oven and let stand for 10 minutes before removing from the pan. Cool on a wire rack.

 *vegetarian*

**Per Serving:** Kcal 147, Protein 3g, Carb 31g, Fat 1g, Sodium 374mg, Dietary Fiber 1g
**Daily Values:** Fiber 5%, Vit C 5%, Vit A 1%, Vit D 1%, Calcium 3%, Iron 5%

*PURPLE CORN RECIPES*

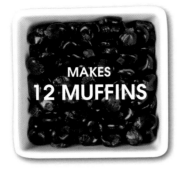

# PURPLE CORN MUFFINS

*This wonderful muffin recipe comes to us from Morena Escardó, the culinary genius behind the blog PeruDelights. We met up with Morena for a three-hour lunch at celebrity chef Gastón Acurio's restaurant, Panchita. After a few rounds of Pisco Sours, she happily agreed to create some traditional Peruvian recipes using a few of our power food ingredients.*

*You won't believe your eyes when you see these muffins. They have a beautiful purple color, with a light and delicious corn flavor, a tender crumb, and some pieces of dried pichuberry. Eat them warm, fresh from the oven. They keep well at room temperature and can be reheated. We love to slice them in half and toast them lightly, and then serve them with honey butter or pichuberry marmalade (see page 33).*

## Ingredients

1¼ cups all-purpose flour

1¼ cups purple corn flour

2¼ teaspoons baking powder

1 teaspoon salt

½ cup dried pichuberry

⅔ cup butter

½ cup sugar

3 eggs

¾ cup buttermilk

## Directions

1. Preheat the oven to 350 degrees F. Grease a 12-cup muffin pan.

2. Sift the flours, baking powder, and salt in a large bowl. Add the dried pichuberries.

3. In another bowl, using an electric mixer, cream the butter with the sugar until pale and fluffy. Add the eggs, one by one, and beat until smooth. Fold the dry ingredients into the butter mixture, alternating with adding the buttermilk; mix lightly until combined.

4. Divide the batter evenly among the muffin cups (an ice cream scoop is perfect for this). Bake for 15 minutes or until well risen. Because the muffins are purple, they won't brown. To see if they are ready, insert a toothpick into a muffin; the toothpick should come out clean with only a few moist crumbs attached to it. Cool the muffins in the pan for a few minutes before serving.

*These muffins keep well for up to three days at room temperature. You can serve them with pichuberry marmalade or with butter whipped with honey.*

PURPLE CORN RECIPES

*vegetarian*

**Per Serving:** Kcal 213, Protein 4g, Carb 23g, Fat 12g, Sodium 235mg, Dietary Fiber 1g
**Daily Values:** Fiber 4%, Vit C 1%, Vit A 16%, Vit D 3%, Calcium 7%, Iron 6%

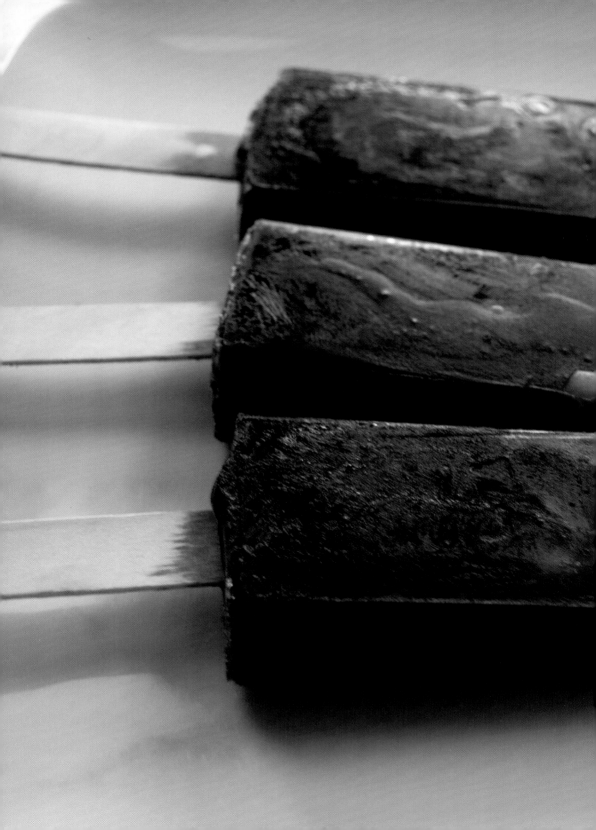

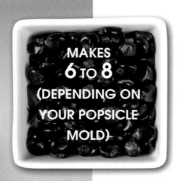

MAKES
**6** TO **8**
(DEPENDING ON
YOUR POPSICLE
MOLD)

# CHICHA MORADA
# PICHUBERRY POPSICLES

*We love the flavor of* chicha morada *so much,
we thought it made sense to freeze it into
Popsicles. And were we ever right—the whole
batch was gone in one afternoon.*

## Ingredients

Chicha morada drink (see page 127)
½ cup pichuberries, halved

## Directions

**1** Pour the chicha morada drink into your Popsicle
molds until they are ¾ of the way full. Add a few halved
pichuberries to each mold. Freeze until firm, about
4 hours or overnight.

PURPLE CORN RECIPES

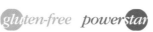

*gluten-free* **powerstar** *vegan*

**Per Serving:** Kcal 119, Protein 1g, Carb 29g, Fat 0g, Sodium 24mg, Dietary Fiber 2g
**Daily Values:** Fiber 8%, Vit C 25%, Vit A 4%, Vit D 4%, Calcium 2%, Iron 2%

# MAZAMORRA MORADA (PURPLE CORN PUDDING)

Mazamorra Morada is a popular Peruvian dessert that shares the same delicately spiced flavor as the chicha morada drink. This is a universal recipe, which we made our own by adding dried pichuberries alongside the prunes.

## Ingredients

1 cup dried fruit (½ cup prune halves and ½ cup dried pichuberries)

1 pound dried purple corn

12 cups water

½ pineapple, chopped into small pieces (reserve the peel)

4 tablespoons cornstarch

3 cinnamon sticks

1 teaspoon whole cloves

1 green apple, peeled and diced

½ cup agave

Pinch of salt

Juice of 1 lime

## Directions

**1** Place the dried prunes and pichuberries in a bowl and cover with about 2 cups of boiling water. Set aside to cool.

**2** Add the purple corn to a large pot and cover with 10 cups water. Add the pineapple peel, cinnamon sticks, and cloves. Bring the water to a boil, and boil uncovered for about 30 minutes, until the liquid is a bright purple color. Strain the liquid and return to pot. Discard the pulp from the strainer.

**3** Remove ½ cup of the purple corn liquid from the pot and transfer it to a small bowl. Stir in the cornstarch until completely mixed and set aside.

**4** Add the dried fruits, pineapple, apple, agave, and a pinch of salt to the large pot of purple corn liquid. Bring the mixture to a boil again, then reduce to simmer for about 20 minutes, stirring occasionally, until the apple is soft. Whisk the cornstarch mixture into the simmering mixture and continue to cook, stirring constantly, for about 5 minutes more or until mixture has thickened. Remove from the heat and stir in the lime juice.

**5** Serve chilled or at room temperature, sprinkled with cinnamon.

PURPLE CORN RECIPES

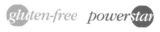 

*gluten-free* **powerstar** *vegan*

**Per Serving:** Kcal 240, Protein 2g, Carb 60g, Fat 1g, Sodium 102mg, Dietary Fiber 4g
**Daily Values:** Fiber 17%, Vit C 56%, Vit A 12%, Vit D 0%, Calcium 4%, Iron 5%

# 9 ⌒ ARTICHOKES

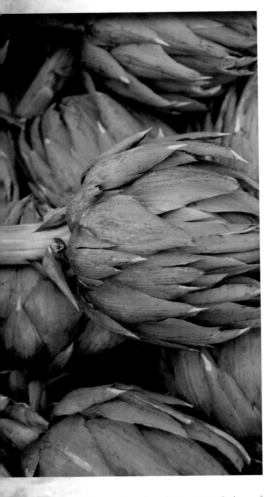

## OVERVIEW

**ARTICHOKES ARE,** of course, a vegetable, but many don't realize that they are part of the sunflower family; they are actually the bud of the plant's flower. The green vegetable is a bundle of tightly layered leaves, which can be peeled back to reveal the tender delicacy known as the artichoke heart.

While there is work involved in eating an artichoke—first navigating the spiny leaves, then cutting the bristles from the heart—the experience is rewarding both from a taste and a health perspective. Studies show that artichokes contain the most antioxidants of any vegetable and they placed seventh in a ranking of 1,000 different antioxidant foods. Some of the most potent antioxidants found in artichokes include quercetin, rutin, anthocyanins, cynarin, luteolin, and silymarin.

Though we often associate artichokes with Mediterranean countries, Peru is actually the third largest exporter of artichokes in the world. And the artichokes that grow there are Amazonian in size and character, with huge leaves and sharp clawlike thorns on the end.

*Artichokes can be steamed or grilled, and eaten on their own—often with a lemon-based aioli or lemon butter. They can also be prepared as a versatile ingredient in pastas, pizzas, stews, and summer salads.*

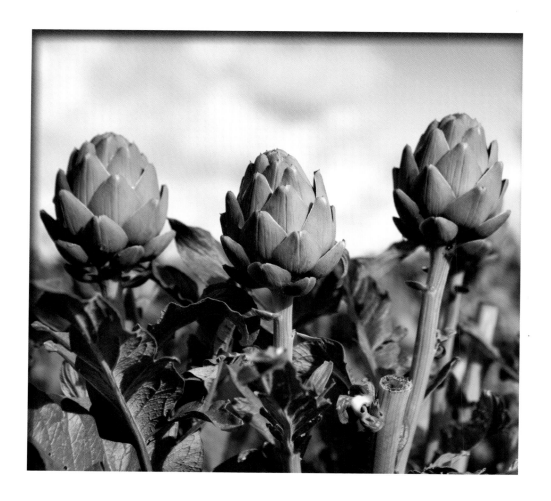

# NUTRITION & HEALTH
## BENEFITS

ANTICANCER

CHOLESTEROL REDUCING

DETOXIFIES

DIABETES FRIENDLY

GUT HEALTHY

HEART HEALTHY

LIVER PROTECTING

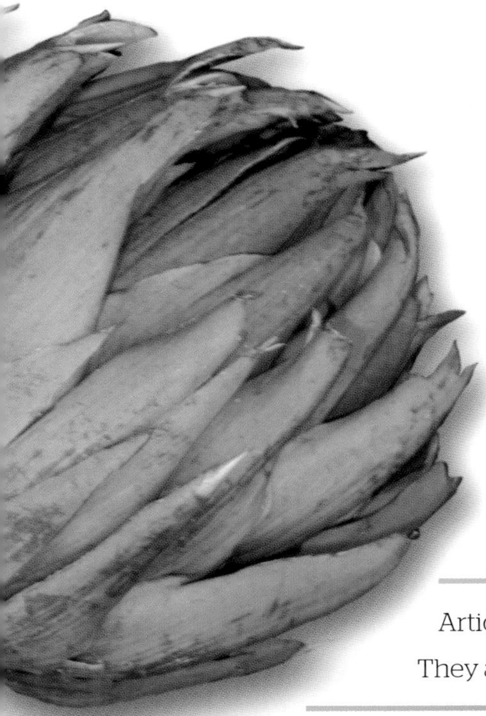

Artichokes are rich in vitamin C, calcium, fiber, and iron. They are low in both fat and calories.

Artichokes help protect liver cells. They contain silymarin, which is a flavonoid that supports liver health. Silymarin has been proven to stimulate cell regeneration and fight harmful free radicals. In this way, it clears some of the toxic load the liver would otherwise have to process.

Artichokes are a great source of dietary fiber, which means they can help lower the risk of developing heart disease, stroke, hypertension, and diabetes. Fiber also improves blood sugar levels and insulin sensitivity in nondiabetic and diabetic individuals.

Increased fiber intake is also helpful in treating gastrointestinal disorders, including acid reflux disease, duodenal ulcer, diverticulitis, constipation, and hemorrhoids.

Artichokes have been proven to lower blood pressure and cholesterol levels.

What's more, artichoke extract reduced the growth and spread of cancer cells, making artichokes a true power food.

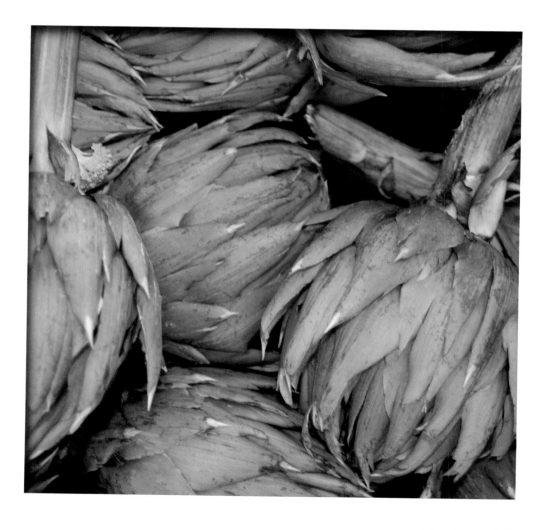

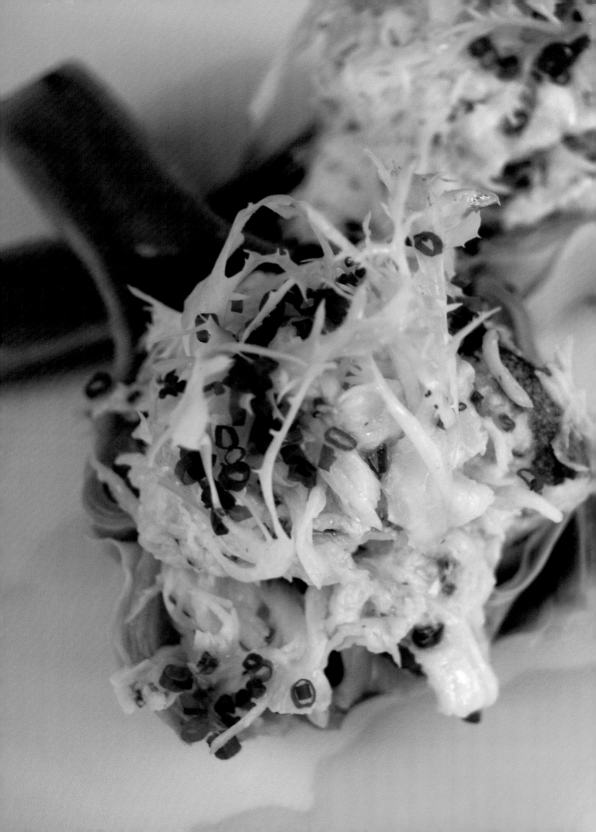

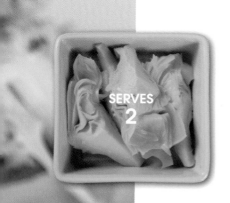

SERVES
2

# STUFFED ARTICHOKE

*When artichokes and crabs are both in season, they make a beautiful flavor pairing. Jason D'Angelo from San Francisco's Waterbar shared this dish, which showcases both delicate flavors in a simple, fresh preparation.*

## Ingredients

2 artichokes

4 ounces crabmeat

2 tablespoon crème fraiche

1 tablespoon lemon zest

1 tablespoon chopped chives

1 teaspoon olive oil

Salt to taste

Frisée to garnish (curly chicory or endive)

## Directions

1. Cover the artichokes with water in a large pot and bring to a boil. Reduce the heat to a simmer and cook for 25 to 45 minutes or until the outer leaves of the artichoke can easily be pulled off. Set aside to cool. Once cooled, cut the artichokes in half and remove the inner choke (or heart) and bristles with a spoon.

2. In a bowl, combine the crabmeat, crème fraiche, lemon zest, chives, and oil. Mix well and season to taste.

3. Stuff each artichoke half with 2 tablespoons of the crabmeat mixture. Plate and garnish with frisée.

**Per Serving:** Kcal 194, Protein 16g, Carb 15g, Fat 9g, Sodium 315mg, Dietary Fiber 8g
**Daily Values:** Fiber 30%, Vit C 42%, Vit A 2%, Vit D 0%, Calcium 13%, Iron 12%

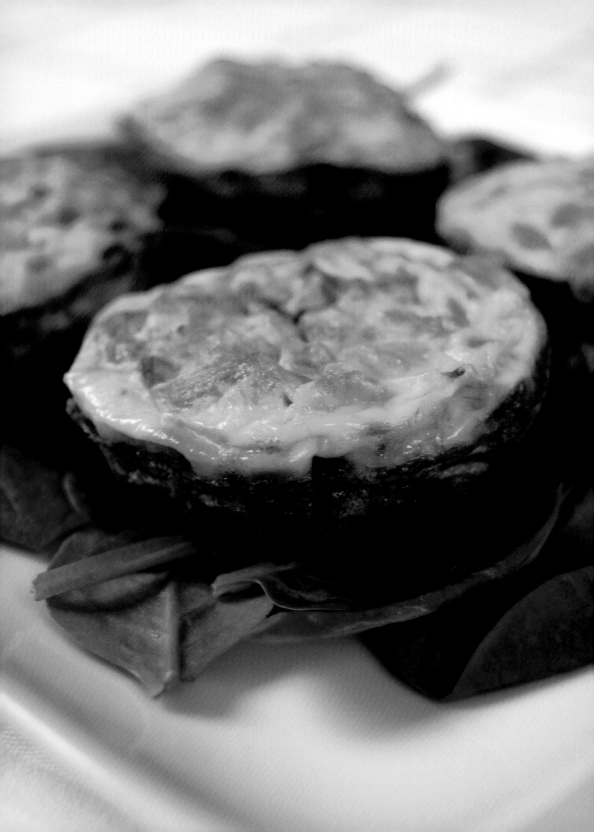

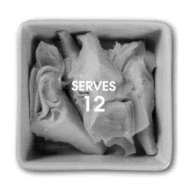

# EGG WHITE AND ARTICHOKE QUINOA MUFFINS

**SERVES 12**

*This is one of our favorite tricks for prepping food for the week. Make these egg white "muffins" on a Sunday and they'll make an easy grab-and-go breakfast for hurried weekday mornings. If you want a little added flavor dimension, feel free to throw in whatever cheese you have on hand: crumbled chevre, feta, or grated Parmesan are all great options.*

## Ingredients

½ cup chopped red onion

1 (14-ounce) can artichoke hearts, drained and chopped

1 tablespoon olive oil

16 ounces egg whites

1 cup cup quinoa

Salt and pepper to taste, approximately 1 teaspoon of each

## Directions

1. Preheat the oven to 350 degrees F.

2. In a frying pan, sauté the onion, artichoke hearts, and oil over medium heat until the onions are soft. Remove from the heat and cool.

3. In a medium bowl, combine the egg whites, quinoa, and cooled vegetable mixture. Add the salt and pepper. Gently fold together.

4. Spray muffin tins with nonstick cooking spray, and transfer the egg mixture to muffin tins using a ¼-cup ladle or measuring cup.

5. Bake on the middle rack for 10 to 15 minutes. To check for doneness, insert a toothpick near the center of a muffin to ensure it comes out clean.

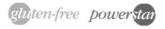 *gluten-free* **powerstar** *vegan*

**Per Serving:** Kcal 66, Protein 6g, Carb 8g, Fat 2g, Sodium 84mg, Dietary Fiber 3g
**Daily Values:** Fiber 13%, Vit C 5%, Vit A 0%, Vit D 0%, Calcium 1%, Iron 3%

**ARTICHOKE RECIPES**

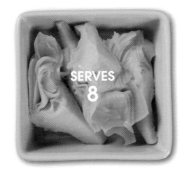

SERVES 8

# ARTICHOKE OLIVE MOUSSE

*This is another classic Peruvian recipe from PeruDelights* chef Morena Cuadra. *She tells us: "Artichokes are found year-round in Peruvian markets, and you can buy them whole, or just the hearts. Either way, they are always fresh and raw. To make this mousse, you can use canned or jarred artichoke hearts to make it easier; just rinse well before using to get rid of the canned taste. And be sure to buy the hearts packed in water, not vinaigrette. Botija or Alfonso olives are perfect for the famous* olivo *sauce, which is usually used in a traditional seafood dish called Pulpo al Olivo."*

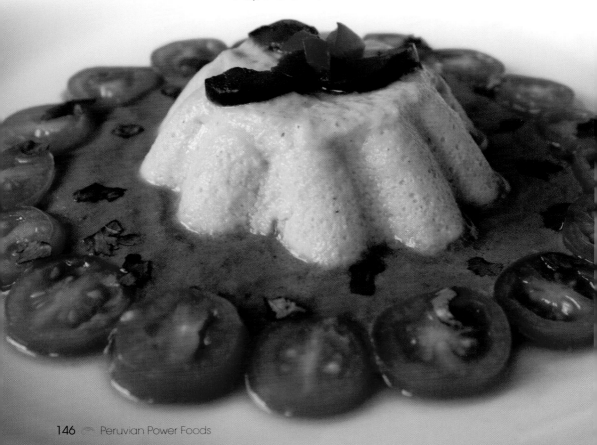

## Ingredients

### For the mousse:

1 cup pureed artichoke hearts
2 eggs
¾ cup cream
¼ teaspoon nutmeg
Salt and pepper to taste
½ cup grated Parmesan cheese
1 handful chopped fresh basil (optional)

### For the olive sauce:

½ cup mayonnaise
¾ cup pitted black olives
1 teaspoon aji paste

## Directions

### For the mousse:

1. Preheat the oven to 350 degrees F.

2. Process the artichoke hearts in a blender to make a puree. Pass the puree through a colander for a smoother mousse.

3. With a hand mixer, beat the eggs, cream, nutmeg, and salt and pepper until creamy. Add the Parmesan cheese and the artichoke puree.

4. Grease a large baking pan or several small ones for individual portions. Pour the artichoke mixture into the pan. Bake in a water bath for 1 hour. (To make a water bath, or bain marie, take a larger casserole dish and fill it halfway with water. Simply place the baking pan or pans into the larger container so the baking pan is surrounded by the water bath.)

### For the sauce:

5. While the artichoke mousse is baking, prepare the olive sauce by blending the mayonnaise, olives, and aji together until smooth.

6. Remove the mousse and cool inside the water bath; unmold while still a bit warm. Serve with the olive sauce on a bed of tomato slices, and sprinkle with chopped basil (optional).

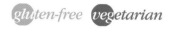 *gluten-free* *vegetarian*

**Per Serving:** Kcal 186, Protein 5g, Carb 7g, Fat 16g, Sodium 333mg, Dietary Fiber 3g
**Daily Values:** Fiber 13%, Vit C 4%, Vit A 8%, Vit D 4%, Calcium 10%, Iron 5%

Artichokes  147

**ARTICHOKE RECIPES**

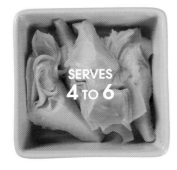

SERVES
4 TO 6

# ARTICHOKE DIP

*Artichokes pair beautifully with cheese, and this makes a wonderful savory dip with toasted pita chips. It's perfect for a cocktail party or an any-time snack. This version uses Neufchatel, which is the lighter, lower-fat version of cream cheese. Please note, this is a versatile dip and you can always toss in a little feta, chevre, or other creamy cheese if you have some in the fridge.*

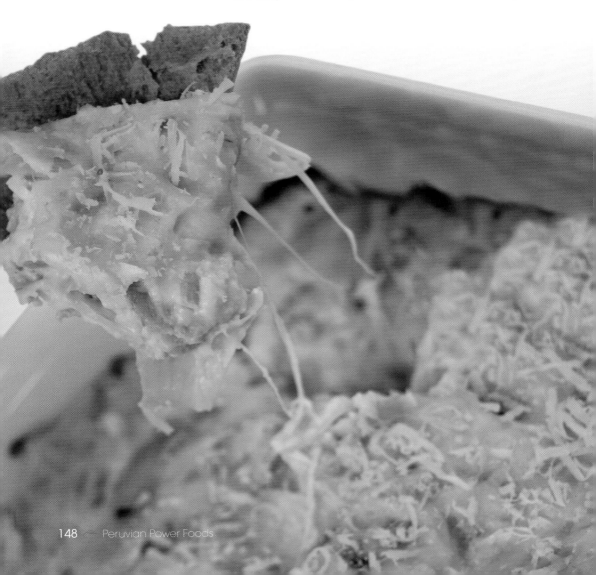

## Ingredients

### For the dip:

2 tablespoons olive oil

1 yellow onion, diced

5 garlic cloves, finely chopped

3 (14-ounce) cans artichoke hearts
packed in water, drained and chopped

5 shakes Tabasco or similar hot sauce

½ cup dry white wine

Salt and pepper to taste

4 ounces Neufchatel cream cheese

2 cups shredded mozzarella

1 cup shredded Parmesan

### For the pita chips:

10 pita bread pockets

¼ cup olive oil

Sea salt to taste

## Directions

1. Preheat the oven to 400 degrees F. In a large skillet, sauté the onion in olive oil until translucent and soft, about 5 minutes. Add the garlic and cook for another 2 minutes, stirring often. Add the artichokes, hot sauce, and wine. Cook down until the wine evaporates, about 5 minutes. Season with salt and pepper.

2. Pull the skillet from the heat and stir in the Neufchatel. Add the mozzarella and incorporate. Transfer the mixture to an 8 x 8 inch baking dish; sprinkle with Parmesan. Bake until golden brown, about 30 minutes.

3. While the dip is baking, cut pita pockets into triangles and split them at the seams. Brush with olive oil and sprinkle with sea salt. Spread them on a cookie sheet and bake at 350 degrees until golden brown, approximately 10 minutes. Serve the pita chips alongside the dip.

**Per Serving:** Kcal 333, Protein 19g, Carb 15g, Fat 21g, Sodium 626mg, Dietary Fiber 7g
**Daily Values:** Fiber 29%, Vit C 14%, Vit A 11%, Vit D 0%, Calcium 51%, Iron 6%

ARTICHOKE RECIPES

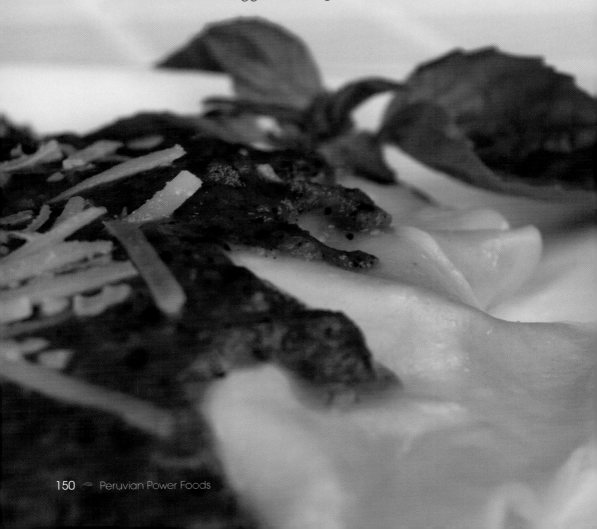

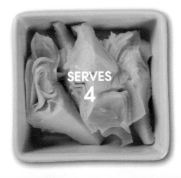

SERVES
4

# ARTICHOKE RAVIOLI WITH ROASTED TOMATO SAUCE

*One of our favorite secrets for making an easy dish that's sure to impress is using wonton wrappers to make ravioli. These wrappers can be easily found in Asian markets, or healthier grocery stores, and once boiled, they make perfect little pasta pockets for any kind of filling. The trick is to use just a little filling, and be sure you pinch and seal them tightly with enough egg wash to "glue" them shut.*

## Ingredients

### For sauce:

4 tablespoons olive oil

8 roma or heirloom tomatoes, whole, or halved if large

1 large red onion, cut into 6 rough pieces

2 red peppers, quartered and seeded

Salt and pepper to taste

### For ravioli:

1 (16-ounce) can or jar artichoke hearts packed in water, chopped

10 3 x 3-inch wonton wrappers (they come in packs of at least 40)

¼ cup grated Parmesan

¼ cup crumbled feta or chevre

2 eggs, beaten (for egg wash)

1 pastry brush

## Directions

**1** Coat a cast-iron skillet with the olive oil over high heat and add the tomatoes, onion, and red peppers, allowing veggies to sear in the pan. Once they are well browned on the outside, turn the burner down to medium heat and continue to cook on the stovetop or in the oven at 350 degrees until all of the veggies are soft and cooked through. Set aside to cool.

**2** In a bowl, mix together the chopped artichokes and cheeses. Place two wonton wrappers in front of you. Using a pastry brush, paint the perimeter of one wrapper with the beaten egg wash. This is the "glue" that will hold the two pieces together. Place a small spoonful of the artichoke and cheese mixture in the center of the wrapper you've brushed. Now lay the other wrapper on top and pinch the edges together, ensuring that the egg wash holds. If it doesn't, you need to add more egg wash. Continue the process to make 10 ravioli.

**3** Bring a large pot of salted water to a boil. While you're waiting for the water to boil, toss all of your roasted veggies in a blender and puree. Add salt and pepper to taste.

**4** Once the water is boiling, gently place 5 ravioli at a time into the water using a slotted spoon. Let the ravioli cook until lightly translucent, like cooked pasta, approximately 1 minute. Remove the first batch of ravioli with a slotted spoon and then cook the remaining 5. Drain well and serve with the pureed roasted tomato sauce.

*vegetarian*

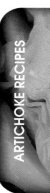

**Per Serving:** Kcal 340, Protein 16g, Carb 45g, Fat 13g, Sodium 449mg, Dietary Fiber 15g
**Daily Values:** Fiber 59%, Vit C 258%, Vit A 46%, Vit D 3%, Calcium 17%, Iron 17%

ARTICHOKE RECIPES

# 10 ⌒ SACHA INCHI

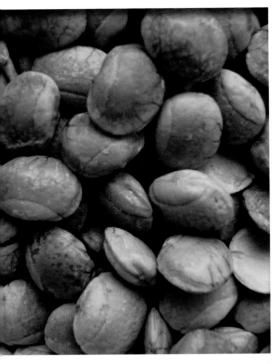

Sacha inchi is known in its native Peru by many names: Inca peanut, wild peanut, Inca inchi, or mountain peanut. But whatever you call it, sacha inchi is a singular power food, providing the highest levels of omega-3 fatty acids in any plant on the planet! It was so cherished in Incan civilization that representations of the plant and its fruits have been found in Incan tombs. Sacha inchi remains a treasured staple in the diet of many native tribal groups in Peru.

## OVERVIEW

**THE SACHA INCHI PLANT** produces star-shaped fruits with dark brown seeds inside that are the size of a macadamia. Despite occasionally being referred to as a peanut, it is not a nut at all, but rather a seed, which can be eaten whole, or pressed to produce an antioxidant-rich oil. A fantastic source of omega-3 and omega-6 oils, as well as vitamin E and serotonin-boosting tryptophan, sacha inchi is a gold mine of essential nutrients. It's also one of the most powerful inflammation fighters ever discovered. The omega-3 contained in sacha inchi is an essential fatty acid for human life that cannot be synthesized from the standard food we eat daily, so we need to ingest it from power sources.

Besides being the oil lowest in saturated fats, sacha inchi is a wonderful resource for pregnant or breast-feeding women seeking safe omega-3s without the mercury risks associated with seafood. By volume, sacha inchi has over 48 percent omega-3s—that's over 84 percent total essential fatty acids. And those highly-concentrated omega-3s fight disease-causing inflammation. Similar to flaxseed oil, it's a food that's naturally perfectly balanced, offering the optimum ratio of omega-3 and omega-6 acids. That's important because the balance between these two types of fatty acids has been proven to decrease risk factors for chronic diseases.

The seeds are loaded with protein at 9 grams per ounce, and rich in tryptophan, an amino acid that's a precursor to the production of serotonin, the important hormone that can help promote a positive mood.

Sacha inchi is truly a power food that brings myriad health benefits to everyone who incorporates it into their regular diet.

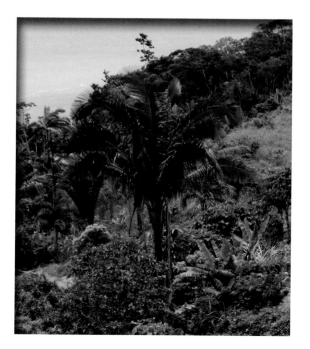

*Sacha inchi is now available in the United States in both the seed and oil forms, which makes it easy to adapt this potent source of essential oils into many kinds of dishes. The seed is wonderful on its own, as a snack, or tossed into salads, energy bars, and the like. The oil can be used in any dish that typically calls for olive oil—in salads, shakes, vegetables, and dips. Please note, sacha inchi should not be heated—its power comes from its raw state, so cooking with it will immediately deplete its omega benefits. Also, like other potent omega oils, it needs to be stored in a cold, dark place to retain optimum freshness. Once opened, follow the guidelines about expiration. In general, the seed and the oil have a pleasant grassy taste.*

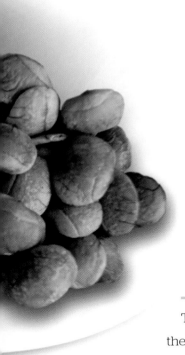

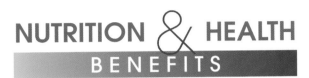

# NUTRITION & HEALTH
## BENEFITS

ANTI-INFLAMMATORY

BRAIN HEALTHY

HEART HEALTHY

SUPPORTS IMMUNE SYSTEM

This oil is primarily composed of unsaturated fatty acids, mostly the omega-3 (alpha-linolenic) and omega-6 (alpha-linoleic) fatty acids. Omega-3 and omega-6 are considered essential because the body is unable to synthesize them. Consuming these fatty acids, primarily omega-3 fatty acids, can prevent diseases such as cancer, coronary heart disease, hypertension, and, potentially, rheumatoid arthritis.

There is a strong link between omega-3 fatty acid consumption and healthy brain function. This is because our brains are 60 percent fat, most of which is an omega-3 called DHA. A deficiency of these oils in humans increases the risk for several brain disorders, such as attention deficit disorder, bipolar disorder, dementia, depression, dyslexia, and schizophrenia.

Omega-3s help prevent blood from clogging by keeping saturated fats mobile in the blood stream. They also help with the fluidity of cellular membranes so that oxygen can flow from red blood cells to the body's tissues.

Studies show that supplementing with omega-3s increases cognition in school-aged children.

Omega-3s reduce arterial and tissue inflammation. This is critical because inflammation is linked to heart disease, type 2 diabetes, rheumatoid arthritis, and other chronic diseases. Research shows that omega-3s may reduce proteins that cause inflammation.

Sacha inchi has a high content of vitamin E. Regular consumption of vitamin E has been linked to decreased risk for developing cardiovascular disease. Vitamin E is an antioxidant that helps fight free radicals, which can cause oxidative damage that leads to conditions such as cardiovascular disease.

Overall, we view sachi inchi as a powerful anti-aging food because it promotes longevity by aiding brain function, postponing cognitive decline, improving mental health and alertness, and boosting various brain functions like memory, intelligence, and thinking.

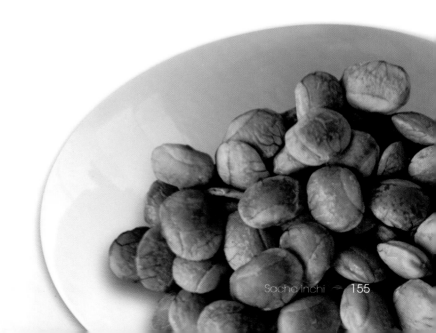

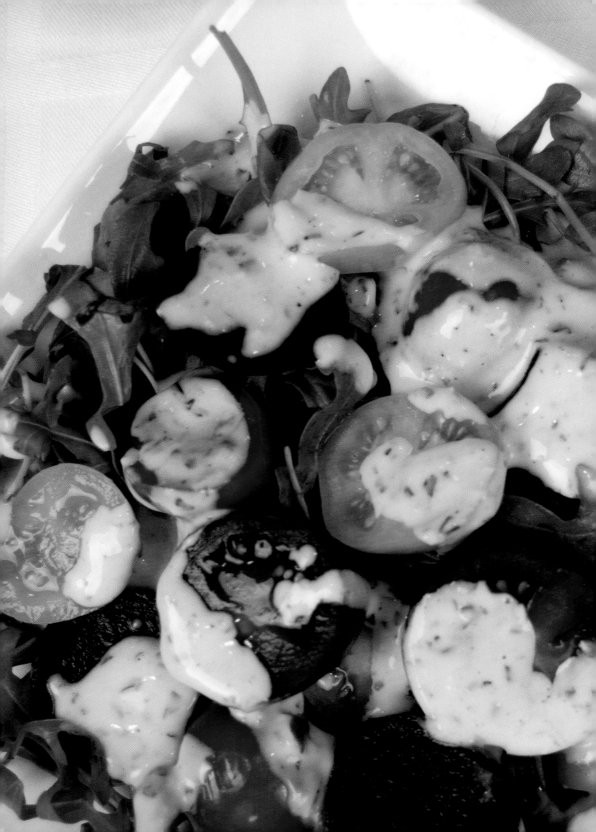

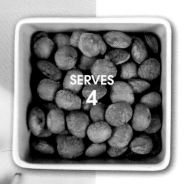

**SERVES 4**

# ZESTY SACHA INCHI CILANTRO DRESSING

*Get all the omega benefits of sacha inchi in a salad dressing just bursting with tangy flavor. You can also drizzle this dressing over roasted veggies, baked chicken, or a baked potato.*

## Ingredients

3 cloves garlic, crushed
⅓ cup lime juice
¼ teaspoon salt
¼ teaspoon pepper
2 tablespoons chopped cilantro
½ cup sacha inchi oil
½ cup nonfat Greek yogurt

## Directions

1. Combine the garlic, lime juice, salt, pepper, and cilantro in a bowl. Slowly whisk the sacha inchi oil into the lime juice mixture until thickened. Whisk the Greek yogurt into the mixture. Refrigerate for 15 minutes or overnight.

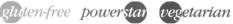 *gluten-free* **powerstar** **vegetarian**

**Per Serving:** Kcal 284, Protein 3g, Carb 4g, Fat 28g, Sodium 157mg, Dietary Fiber 0g
**Daily Values:** Fiber 1%, Vit C 12%, Vit A 1%, Vit D 0%, Calcium 1%, Iron 1%

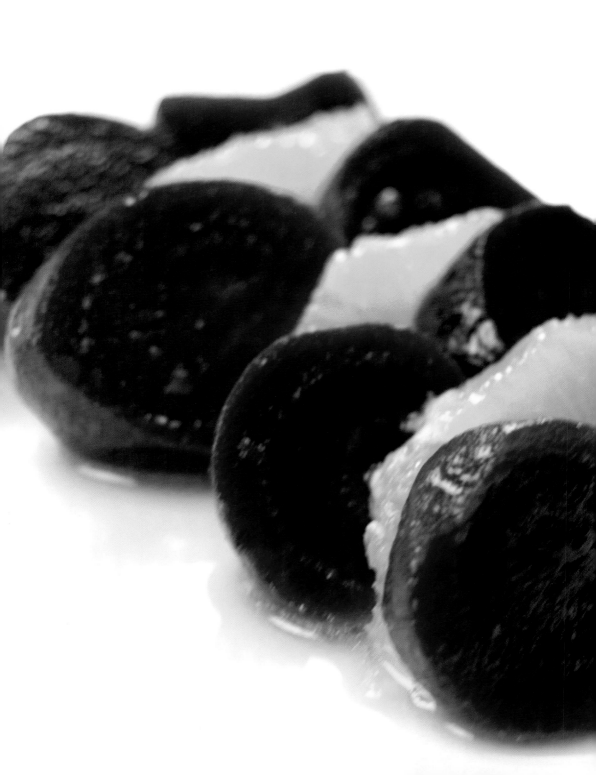

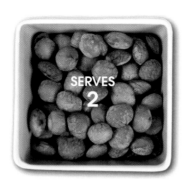

# ORANGE AND BEET SALAD WITH SACHA INCHI DRESSING

*Here, the grassy flavor of sacha inchi oil balances the sweetness of the beets and the citrus notes of the orange segments. This dish became an instant favorite in our summer salad repertoire.*

## Ingredients

4 to 5 medium beets
1 orange, peeled and sliced
Juice of one orange

Juice of one lemon
1 tablespoon sacha inchi oil
1 tablespoon olive oil

## Directions

1. Clean, peel, and cook the beets until soft, boiling them 30–45 minutes depending on the size. Remove the beets from the heat and allow to cool.

2. Once the beets are at room temperature, slice them into rounds. Slice one of the oranges into rounds as well. Arrange the slices on your plate, alternating a beet slice and an orange slice.

3. In a medium bowl, mix the juice from the orange and lemon. Add the sacha inchi oil and season to taste. Drizzle the dressing over the beets and oranges. Enjoy!

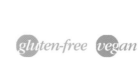

*gluten-free* *vegan*

Per Serving: Kcal 257, Protein 4g, Carb 31g, Fat 14g, Sodium 145mg, Dietary Fiber 7g
Daily Values: Fiber 28%, Vit C 119%, Vit A 6%, Vit D 0%, Calcium 6%, Iron 10%

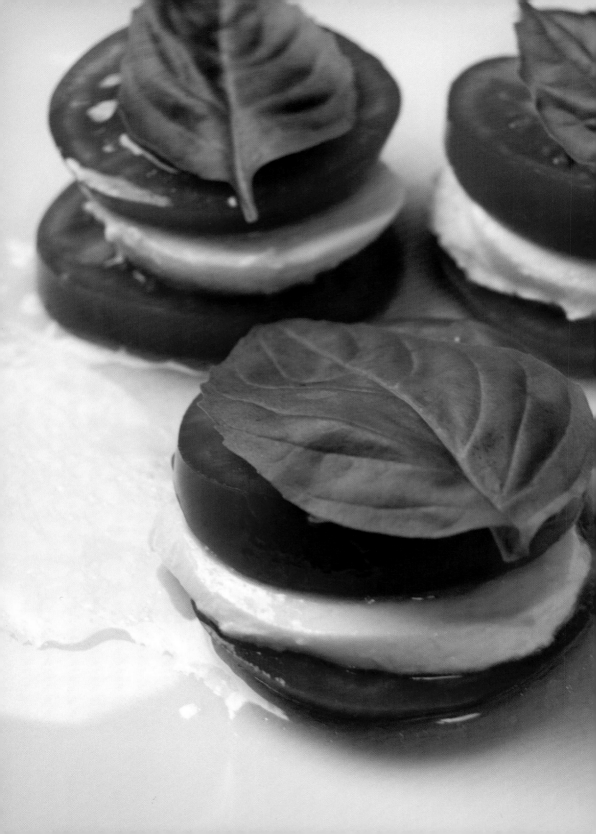

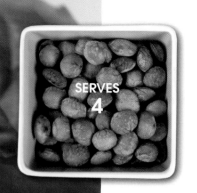

# CAPRESE SALAD WITH SACHA INCHI OIL

*A Mediterranean classic gets a power food makeover with sacha inchi oil replacing the traditional drizzle of olive oil. We love the way the grassy flavor brings out the sweetness of the tomatoes and complements the mozzarella.*

**SERVES 4**

## Ingredients

3 to 4 large tomatoes
4 ounces fresh mozzarella cheese
1 bunch fresh basil
2 tablespoons sacha inchi oil
Salt and pepper to taste

## Directions

1. Slice the tomatoes, discarding the ends. Cut the mozzarella into 2- to 3-inch round slices. Remove eight basil leaves from the stems.

2. On each of 4 plates, stack the salad with one slice of tomato, a basil leaf, one slice of mozzarella cheese, one slice of tomato, and top with a basil leaf. Garnish with a drizzle of sacha inchi oil. Season with salt and pepper.

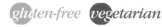

*gluten-free* *vegetarian*

Per Serving: Kcal 168, Protein 9g, Carb 6g, Fat 12g, Sodium 156mg, Dietary Fiber 2g
Daily Values: Fiber 6%, Vit C 28%, Vit A 29%, Vit D 0%, Calcium 23%, Iron 3%

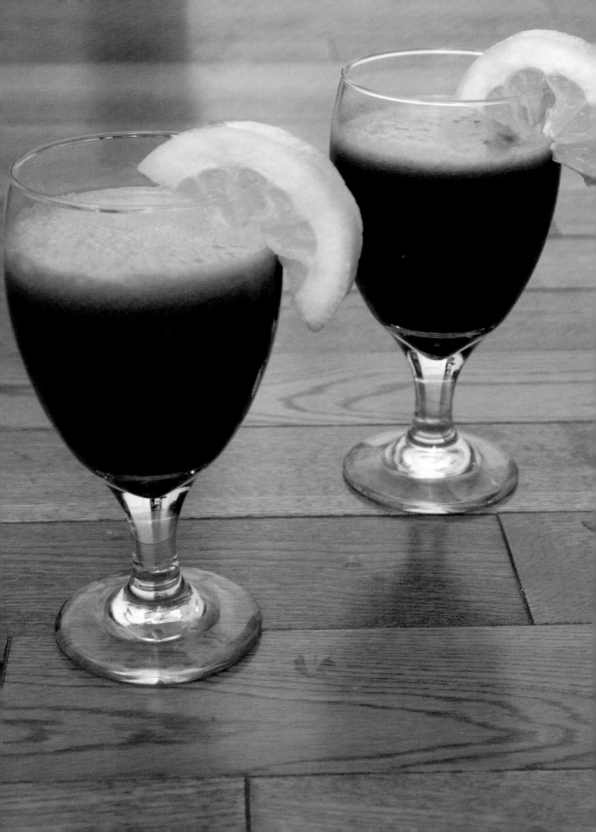

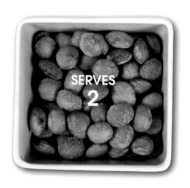

**SERVES 2**

# SUPERGREEN SACHA SMOOTHIE

*This superbooster comes to us from superblogger Morena Escardó from* PeruDelights. *Green juice is gaining in popularity among the health set. By adding two of our Peruvian power-foods—sacha inchi oil and maca—this elixir goes from good to great.*

## Ingredients

1 cucumber

2 celery sticks

4 lettuce leaves

4 spinach leaves

4 chard leaves

4 kale leaves

1 green apple

2 cups chopped pineapple

1-inch piece of fresh ginger

1 tablespoon sacha inchi oil

1 tablespoon maca powder

2 teaspoons sesame seeds

Optional: tablespoon of
    honey or agave

## Directions

**1** Wash, peel, and cut the vegetables and fruits into chunks. (If they're organic, the apple, cucumber, and ginger don't need to be peeled). Juice the vegetables and fruit in your juicer.

**2** Transfer the mixture to a blender, add the sacha inchi oil, maca, and sesame seeds, and blend well. If more sweetness is desired, add honey or agave to taste.

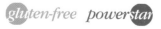 *gluten-free* *powerstar*  *vegan*

Per Serving: Kcal 396, Protein 5g, Carb 79g, Fat 9g, Sodium 67mg, Dietary Fiber 8g
Daily Values: Fiber 31%, Vit C 89%, Vit A 80%, Vit D 0%, Calcium 16%, Iron 15%

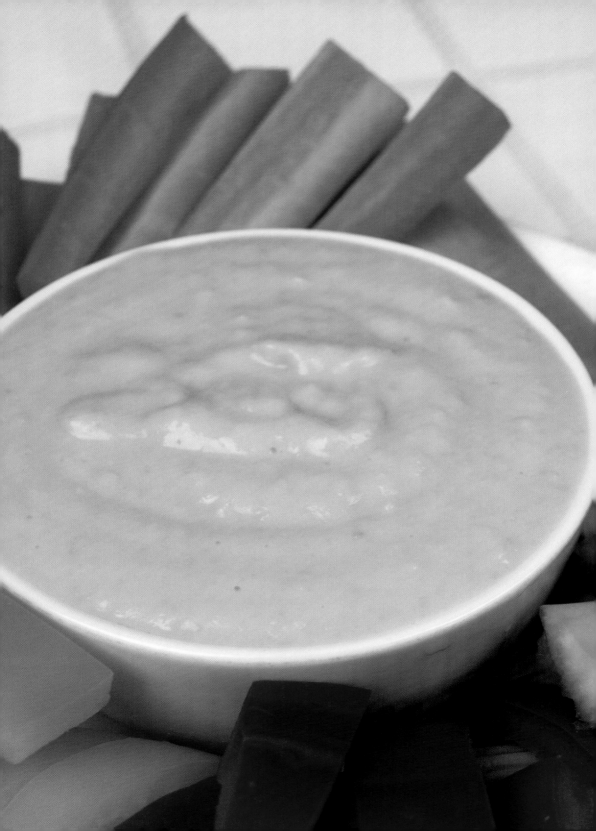

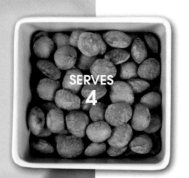

**SERVES 4**

# WHITE BEAN HUMMUS

*This is one of the first recipes we created and it remains one of our go-to favorites. It couldn't be easier to make, and the sacha inchi oil gives it a greater depth of flavor than regular olive oil. It's great as a dip for veggies and toasted pita triangles or as an appetizer at your next social event.*

## Ingredients

1 (16-ounce) can cannellini beans or other white beans, drained and rinsed, reserving 2 tablespoons of the drained liquid

2 tablespoons water or bean liquid

1 clove garlic

1 tablespoon sacha inchi oil

1 tablespoon lemon juice

2 pinches salt

## Directions

**1** In blender or food processor, puree the beans, water or reserved bean liquid, garlic, oil, lemon juice, and salt. Blend until smooth. Store in an airtight container in your refrigerator for up to one week.

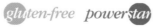 *gluten-free* **powerstar**  *vegan*

**Per Serving:** Kcal 192, Protein 11g, Carb 29g, Fat 4g, Sodium 152mg, Dietary Fiber 7g
**Daily Values:** Fiber 29%, Vit C 3%, Vit A 0%, Vit D 0%, Calcium 10%, Iron 23%

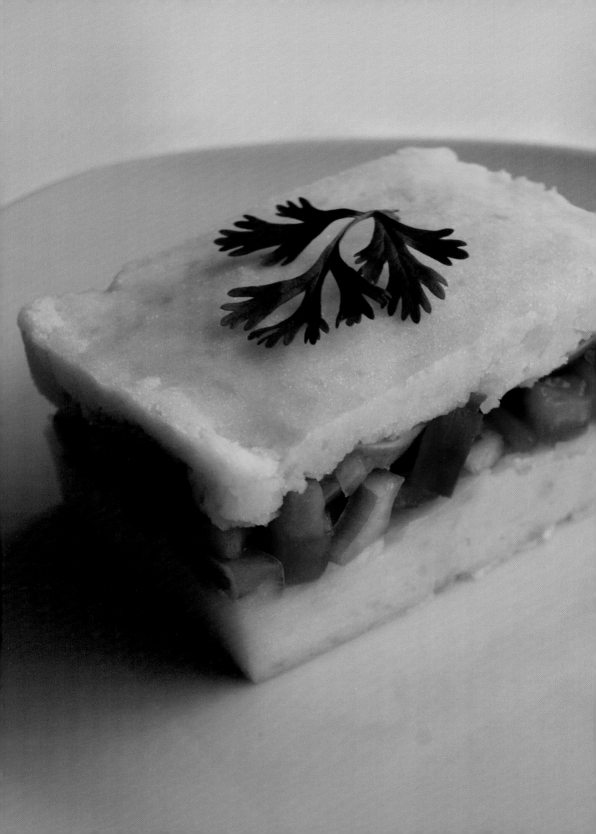

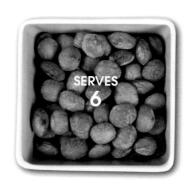

SERVES 6

# VEGGIE CAUSA

*Pronounced* kow-suh, *this potato dish is a traditional favorite in Peru, particularly in Lima and Amazonian areas. Causa is made by using mashed potato to encase any number of fillings, from chicken to fish to sautéed veggies. Here, we've layered the causa to show the filling inside, but it's often served like a potato sandwich, with the filling in the center.*

## Ingredients

2 pounds yellow potatoes

2 tablespoons sacha inchi oil

2 tablespoons aji paste

Juice of 2 limes

Salt and pepper to taste

½ cup cubed onion

1 red bell pepper, chopped into squares

3 tomatoes, chopped into cubes

2 avocados, sliced

Parsley leaves, for garnish

## Directions

1. Cook the potatoes in salted water until they are soft, about 20 to 25 minutes. When cool enough to handle, put through a potato ricer or peel the potatoes and mash them by hand. Mix the potatoes with sacha oil, aji paste, lime juice, and salt and pepper.

2. In separate bowl, mix together the onion, bell pepper, tomatoes, and avocados.

3. Divide the mashed potatoes into two portions. Press one potato portion onto the bottom of a plate. Spoon the vegetable mixture over the top of this potato layer, cover with the second portion of potato, and garnish with parsley leaves.

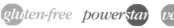 *gluten-free* ***powerstar***  *vegan*

**Per Serving:** Kcal 290, Protein 4g, Carb 42g, Fat 12g, Sodium 24mg, Dietary Fiber 5g
**Daily Values:** Fiber 20%, Vit C 111%, Vit A 24%, Vit D 0%, Calcium 3%, Iron 21%

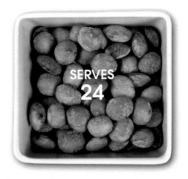

**SERVES 24**

# SACHA INCHI SEED AND KIWICHA GRANOLA

*Talk about power foods. This granola packs protein, antioxidants, whole grains, and fruits for an everyday energy booster that tastes great. Once you've learned how easy it is to make, you'll never want to go back to store-bought again!*

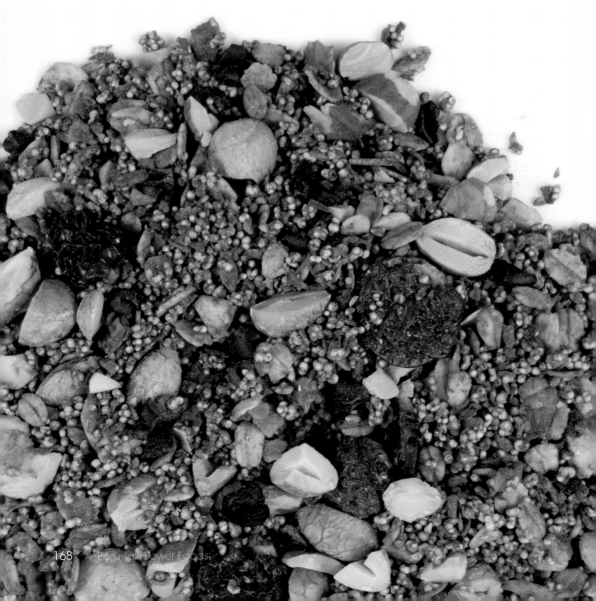

## Ingredients

1 cup old-fashioned oats

2 cups kiwicha, popped
 (see page 73)

½ cup unsweetened shredded
 coconut

1 teaspoon ground cinnamon

½ teaspoon salt

¼ cup lucuma powder

2 tablespoons coconut oil

4 tablespoons honey

½ cup sacha inchi seeds,
 coarsely chopped

½ cup dried pichuberries

½ cup cacao nibs

## Directions

**1** Preheat the oven to 300 degrees F.

**2** In a large bowl, combine the oats, kiwicha, coconut, cinnamon, salt, and lucuma powder.

**3** In a medium saucepan, heat the coconut oil and honey over medium-low heat until smooth.

**4** Add the liquid mixture to the dry ingredients and fold until evenly incorporated.

**5** Place the mixture on a parchment-lined cookie sheet and bake until golden brown, stirring every 10 minutes, roughly 30 minutes.

**6** Cool to room temperature and add the sacha inchi seeds, pichuberries, and cacao nibs. Store in an airtight container at room temperature for up to a week.

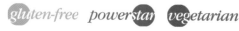 
*gluten-free* *powerstar* *vegetarian*

Per Serving: Kcal 116, Protein 3g, Carb 15g, Fat 5g, Sodium 53mg, Dietary Fiber 3g
Daily Values: Fiber 13%, Vit C 1%, Vit A 4%, Vit D 0%, Calcium 1%, Iron 4%

# 11 ⌒ LUCUMA

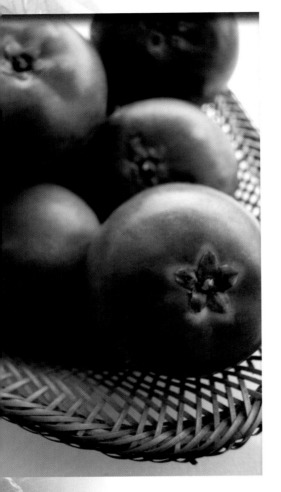

Lucuma is a popular ingredient in many Peruvian desserts, though none more so than ice cream. From the upscale *heladerias* in Lima to corner ice cream stands in Iquitos, lucuma is always a featured, favorite flavor.

## OVERVIEW

**LUCUMA IS A SUBTLY** flavored tropical fruit that grows in the coastal highlands and valleys of Peru.

The flesh of the fruit is a light orange color similar to a persimmon, with a sweet fragrance and surprising, pleasing flavor. Long prized by the native people, it was referred to as the Gold of the Incas. Not only is it dense with nutrients, it's also a versatile ingredient with mild sweetness that lends itself to countless dessert dishes. Depending on its application and degree of sweetness, the flavor profile has been compared to caramel, pumpkin, and maple.

Despite its natural sweetness, lucuma has a very low glycemic index of 25, making it a safe and recommended sweetener for diabetics. Besides adding sweetness, lucuma is a gluten-free antioxidant brimming with fiber, carbohydrates, vitamins, and minerals.

While the fruit is found commonly in South American markets, we see it mostly in powdered form in the United States. For that reason, it's a good idea to think about recipes in which the powder can first be incorporated with warm milk or the like so the grainy texture can be blended to smoothness.

*Because of its mild sweetness and slight maple flavor, lucuma lends itself to dessert dishes. It can be the focal flavor in ice creams, cakes, puddings, and cookies, or it can be added to smoothies, hot cereals, and drinks for a subtle power-food boost.*

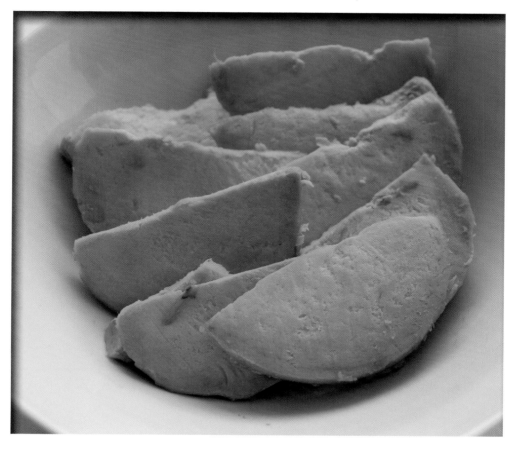

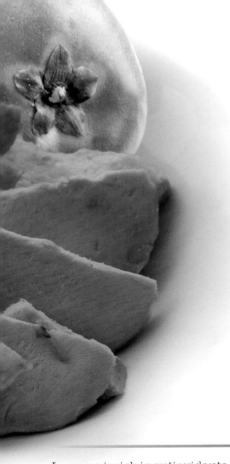

# NUTRITION & HEALTH
## BENEFITS

ANTICANCER

ANTI-INFLAMMATORY

HEART HEALTHY

HELPS CONTROL DIABETES

LOW GLYCEMIC INDEX

PROMOTES SKIN HEALTH

SUPPORTS IMMUNE SYSTEM

Lucuma is rich in antioxidants, fiber, minerals, and vitamins. It also has a good amount of beta-carotene, calcium, flavonoids, iron, magnesium, phosphorus, potassium, and vitamin $B_3$, as well as 14 essential trace elements.

Lucuma helps prevent postprandial hyperglycemia, which suggests that it may help control diabetes.

Studies show lucuma has an impressive anti-inflammatory effect on wound healing and skin aging. Lucuma fatty acids markedly increase wound closure and promote tissue regeneration.

A natural sweetener with a very low glycemic index of 25, lucuma is a safe alternative for diabetics.

Lucuma powder has proven to help control blood pressure.

Lucuma is high in antioxidant-rich, free-radical scavengers called flavonoids. These naturally occurring nutrients have been shown to help prevent coronary heart disease and cancer.

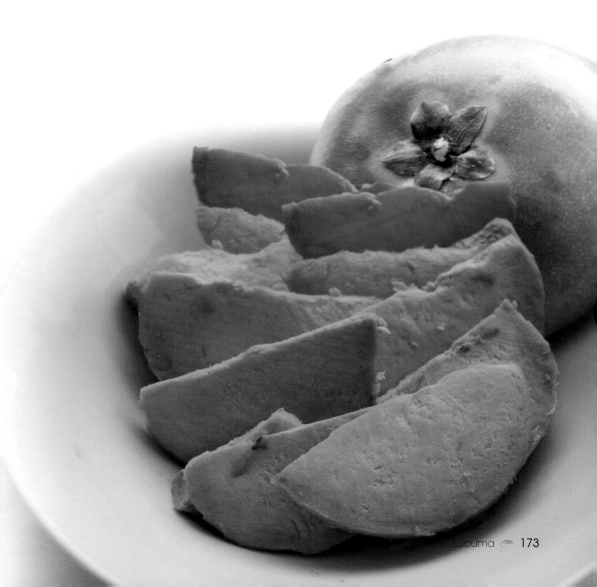

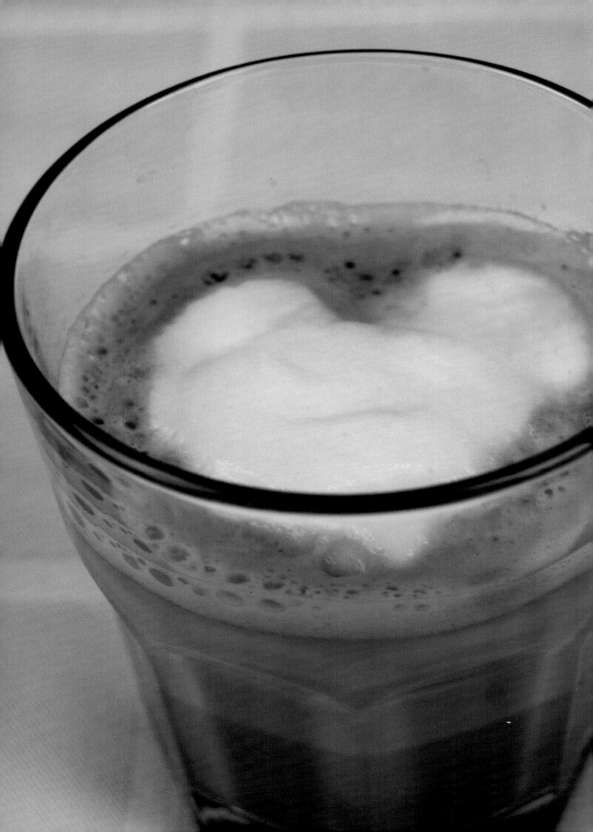

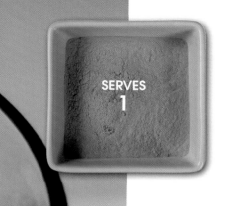

# LUCUMA CAFÉ CON LECHE

**SERVES 1**

*Lucuma has such a deep rich taste, we knew it would pair well in a coffee drink. It gives this drink a hint of cozy maple flavor and a hit of antioxidant power.*

## Ingredients

1 shot espresso
1 teaspoon of agave
2 tablespoons lucuma powder
¼ cup milk
Optional: Milk frother

## Directions

1. Brew one shot of espresso, pour into a mug, and stir in the agave.

2. Dilute the lucuma in a saucepan of warm milk over low heat, or add the lucuma to milk in a warming frother. You may also stir the lucuma into the hot coffee if you prefer—the point is to just use some heat to break down the powder. Pour warm or frothed milk over the coffee and enjoy.

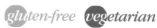 *gluten-free* *vegetarian*

**Per Serving:** Kcal 171, Protein 4g, Carb 35g, Fat 1g, Sodium 43mg, Dietary Fiber 0g
**Daily Values:** Fiber 0%, Vit C 0%, Vit A 2%, Vit D 8%, Calcium 7%, Iron 4%

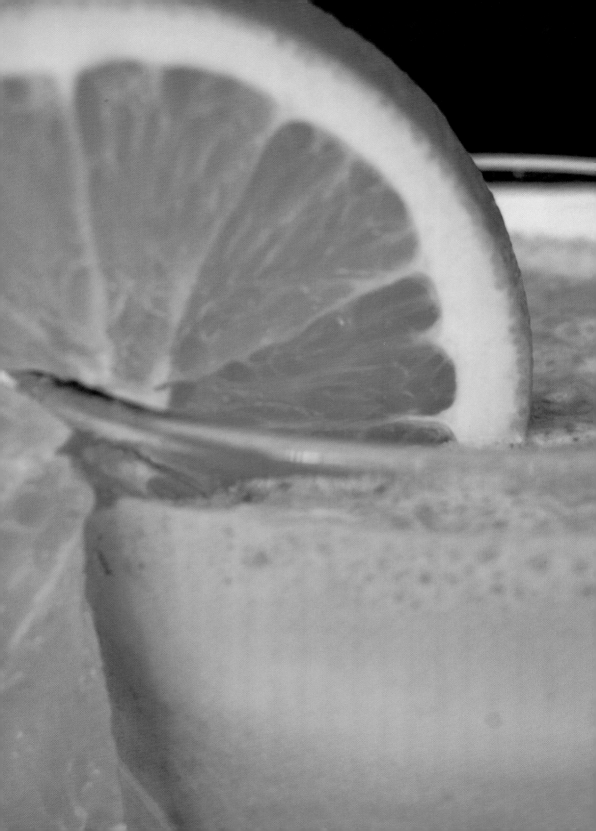

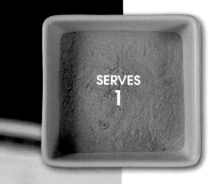

# ORANGE LUCUMA SMOOTHIE

*The combination of orange and lucuma creates a unique flavor blend that is both refreshing and satisfying.*

## Ingredients

2 tablespoons lucuma powder
½ cup orange juice
½ teaspoon vanilla extract
½ cup milk of choice
Handful of ice

## Directions

 Combine all of the ingredients in a blender and mix until smooth.

**LUCUMA RECIPES**

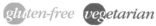 *gluten-free*  *vegetarian*

**Per Serving:** Kcal 233, Protein 7g, Carb 45g, Fat 1g, Sodium 72mg, Dietary Fiber 0g
**Daily Values:** Fiber 1%, Vit C 103%, Vit A 10%, Vit D 16%, Calcium 17%, Iron 6%

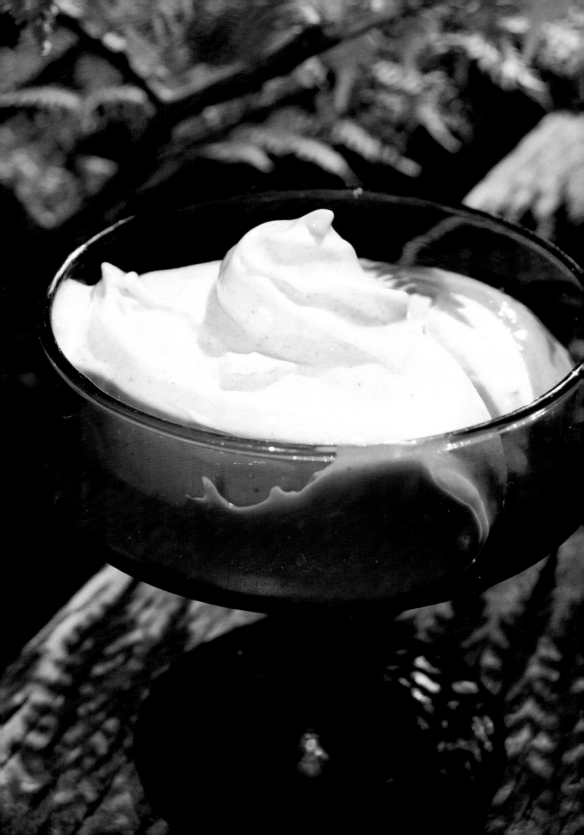

# LUCUMA ICE CREAM

*Lucuma is the most popular ice cream flavor in all of Peru, and it's easy to see why. The unique flavor is reminiscent of maple with a mild sweetness unlike anything else. We found that lucuma in powdered form works just as well as fruit pulp for this recipe and even adds a nice textural grain to the ice cream.*

**SERVES 6**

## Ingredients

1½ cups evaporated milk
8 egg yolks
1 cup sugar

½ cup lucuma powder
1 teaspoon vanilla
2 cups whipping cream

## Directions

**1** Place the evaporated milk in a pot on medium heat. While the evaporated milk is heating to a boil, beat the egg yolks with the sugar until thickened and pale yellow in color.

**2** When the milk reaches a boil, pour a small amount into the egg yolk mixture while whisking. Add the rest of the hot milk and mix well.

**3** Return the hot milk and egg yolk mixture to the pot, and cook on medium-low heat. Cook until the mixture starts to thicken and just barely comes to a boil, stirring constantly. Strain into a clean bowl, and then place bowl in an ice bath.

**4** Add the lucuma powder, vanilla, and whipping cream and mix well. Chill thoroughly. Freeze according to your ice-cream machine manufacturer's directions.

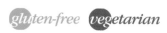

**Per Serving:** Kcal 602, Protein 11g, Carb 61g, Fat 36g, Sodium 112mg, Dietary Fiber 0g
**Daily Values:** Fiber 0%, Vit C 3%, Vit A 26%, Vit D 31%, Calcium 25%, Iron 7%

LUCUMA RECIPES

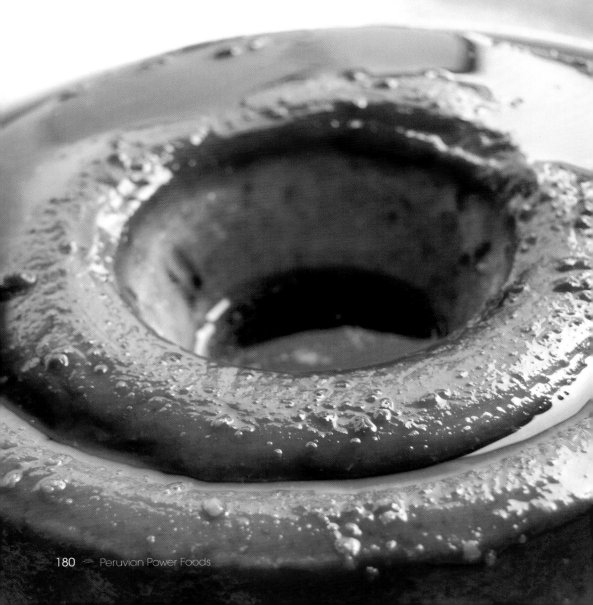

# LUCUMA FLAN

*Flan is a popular dessert across most of South America, and because of its mild flavor, it's the perfect vehicle for some added lucuma flavor. This version comes to us from Manuel's cousin, pastry chef Natahli Giha.*

## Ingredients

### For the caramel:
½ cup granulated sugar
1 fluid ounce water
Bowl of ice water

### For the flan:
1 cup fresh milk
¼ cup white sugar
9 ounces lucuma powder
2 egg yolks
1 whole egg
Pinch of vanilla

## Directions

### For caramel:

1. Preheat the oven to 300 degrees F. Cook the sugar and water over low heat until melted, then increase the heat to high until the mixture is a caramel color. Immerse the pot immediately in an ice water bath to stop cooking.

2. Pour the caramel mixture into a baking dish, ensuring that the caramel covers the bottom and sides. Set aside and allow to cool.

### For flan:

3. Mix together the milk and half of the sugar in another pan and bring to a boil. Remove from the heat. Add the lucuma powder and mix well until incorporated. Add the yolks, whole egg, and remaining sugar, and, finally, the vanilla.

4. Gradually add the boiled milk to the egg mixture, stirring constantly. Strain.

5. Pour the mixture into small molds or ramekins and place them in a water bath or bain marie (fill a Pyrex baking dish ⅔ of the way with hot water). Bake for 60 minutes or until a knife inserted into the center of the flan comes out clean.

LUCUMA RECIPES

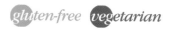

*gluten-free* *vegetarian*

**Per Serving:** Kcal 315, Protein 6g, Carb 64g, Fat 3g, Sodium 48mg, Dietary Fiber 0g
**Daily Values:** Fiber 0%, Vit C 0%, Vit A 4%, Vit D 8%, Calcium 6%, Iron 7%

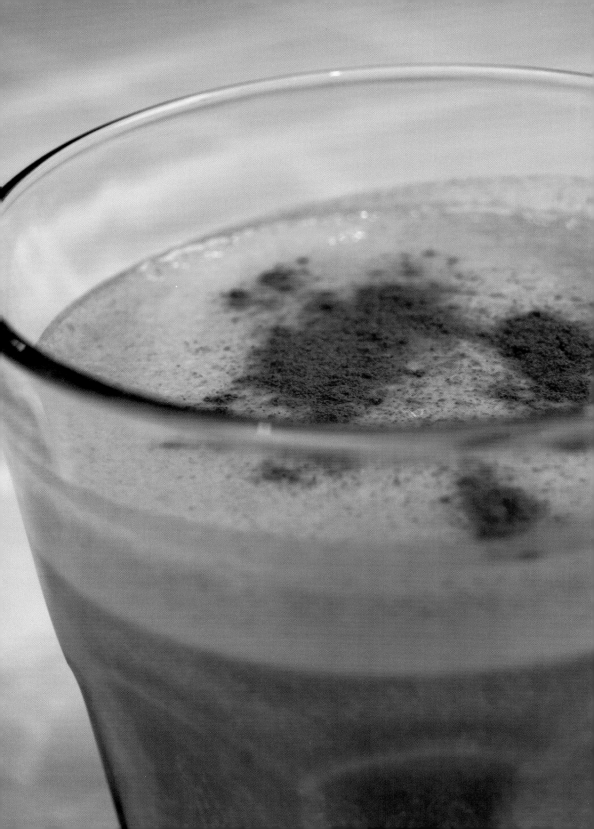

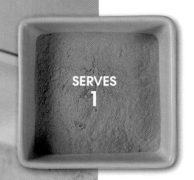

# LUCUMA MILK PISCO

*We love the idea of integrating power foods into delicious cocktails as well as more health-conscious recipes. This frothy "milkshake" is packed with flavor— and punch.*

## Ingredients

2 ounces pisco
2 ounces milk
4 teaspoons lucuma powder
Handful of ice cubes
Sprinkle of cinnamon

## Directions

1  Combine all of the ingredients in a blender and mix until smooth. Garnish with a sprinkle of cinnamon.

 **LUCUMA RECIPES**

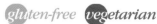 gluten-free  vegetarian

**Per Serving:** Kcal 220, Protein 3g, Carb 25g, Fat 1g, Sodium 34mg, Dietary Fiber 0g
**Daily Values:** Fiber 1%, Vit C 0%, Vit A 2%, Vit D 8%, Calcium 8%, Iron 3%

# 12 ⁀ BEANS

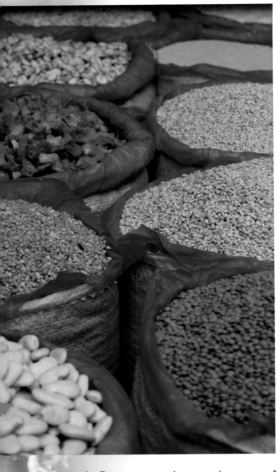

In Peru, *menestras* are bean stews and soups (like the Italian minestrone), which are very popular in home cooking. Almost every mother, regardless of social class and training, has a menestra family recipe in her collection, and every child can recall eating these hearty stews and soups while growing up.

## OVERVIEW

**BEANS ARE AN AGE-OLD PART** of the Peruvian diet. The most commonly found beans are black, canary, fava, and lima beans.

Beans are wonderfully nutritious—full of protein and disease-fighting compounds—but many people are hesitant to eat them because of the potential for intestinal upset. The reason beans can cause gas is because they include a sugar called raffinose, which is also a fiber that we can't digest. But here's a tip: soak the beans for four hours or overnight, and the indigestible sugar will be pulled out of the beans, into the water. You can discard that water, then bring the beans to a boil in a new pot of water for one minute, then drain and discard the water once more. Now you can cook the beans as usual, with fresh water or another cooking liquid, for another hour, or until the beans are done. Going through this extra step will make the beans easily digestible without any unpleasant side effects.

Beans are wonderful on their own or used in soups and side salads. We like making a large amount at the beginning of the week and using them as a go-to protein source tossed into quinoa dishes, served in tacos, added to soups, and more.

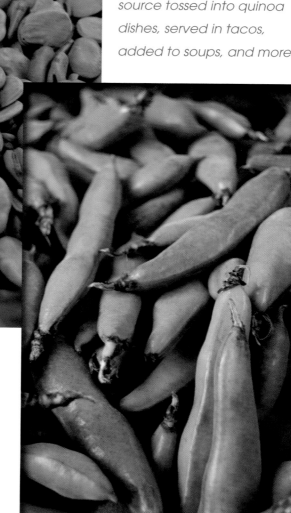

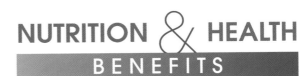

# NUTRITION & HEALTH

ANTICANCER

GUT HEALTHY

HEART HEALTHY

HELPS CONTROL DIABETES

LOWERS CHOLESTEROL

Beans are rich in fiber, folate, iron, magnesium, potassium, protein, and thiamine. Beans are also low in fat.

A diet rich in fiber can significantly lower the risk of developing diabetes, certain gastrointestinal diseases, heart disease, hypertension, obesity, and stroke.

Beans can lower blood pressure and serum cholesterol levels.

Fiber improves blood sugar levels and insulin sensitivity in non-diabetic and diabetic individuals. Fiber can also significantly enhance weight loss efforts.

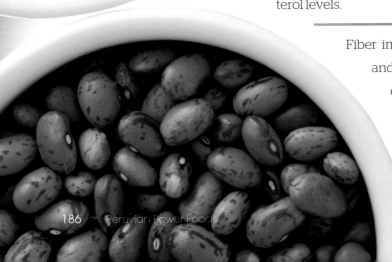

Increased fiber
intake also benefits
a number of gastrointesti-
nal disorders, including acid reflux
disease, constipation, diverticulitis, duodenal ulcer, and hemorrhoids.

Legumes contain compounds that bolster the immune
system to protect against cancers, lower cholesterol levels, and lower blood glucose response.

Beans are rich in iron, so they help to prevent iron-
deficiency anemia, the most common cause of
anemia.

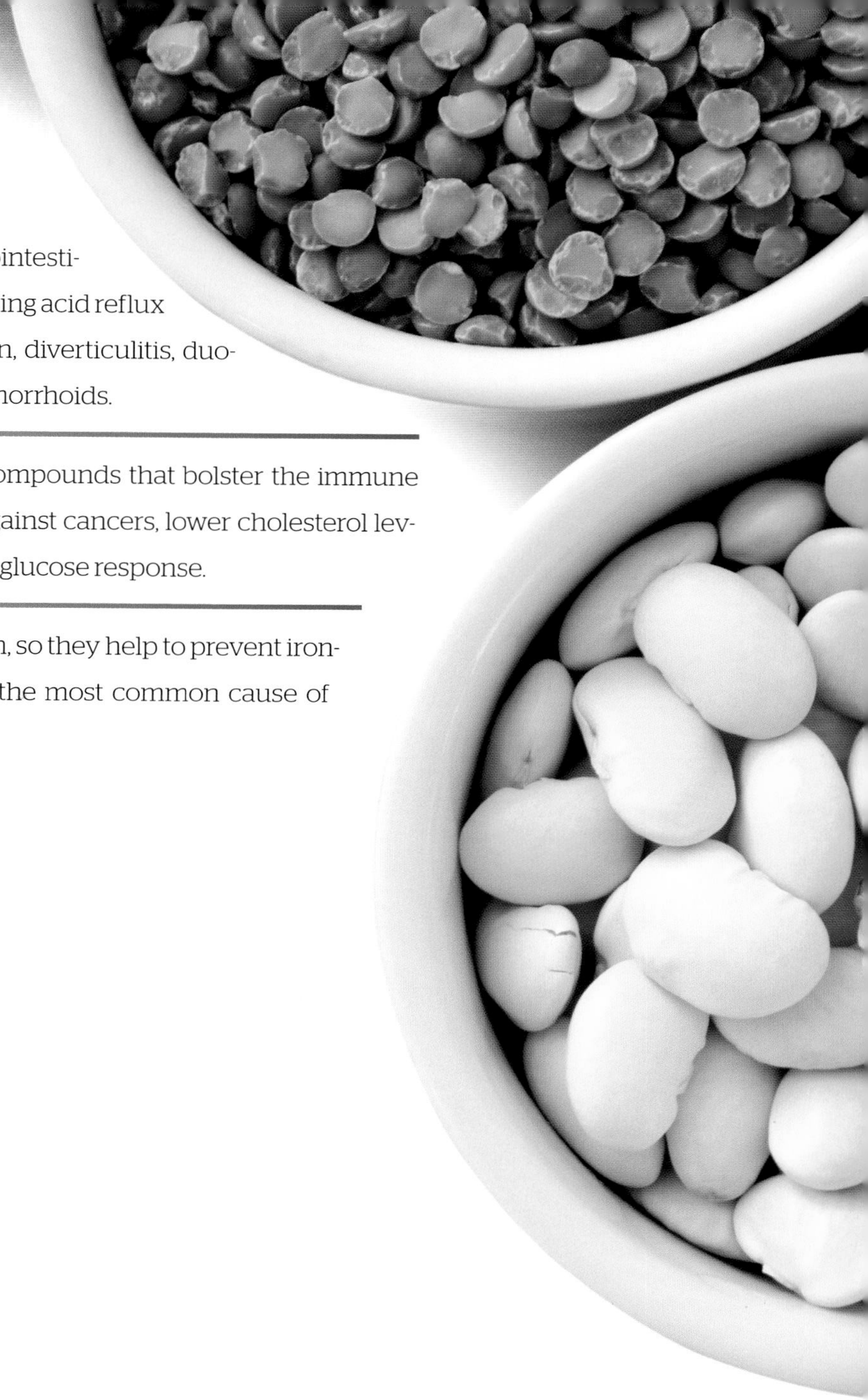

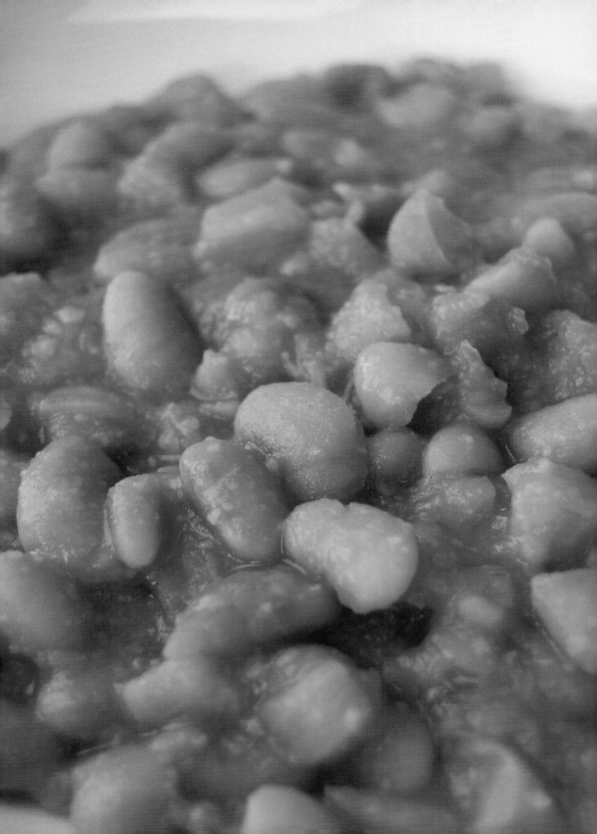

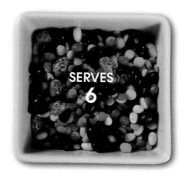

# PERUVIAN STYLE CANARY BEANS

*One of the best things about beans is that they provide plenty of protein, and when prepared with some spice and garlic, they are filling and flavorful enough to make a stand-alone meal.*

## Ingredients

1 pound canary beans

32 ounces vegetable broth

2 tablespoons olive oil

1 medium red onion, chopped

2 teaspoons garlic, crushed

1 tablespoon aji sauce

1 tablespoon tomato paste

Salt and pepper to taste

## Directions

1  Soak the beans for four hours, and then discard the water. Place the beans in a pot with enough water to cover them and bring to boil. Boil for about one minute. Drain the beans and discard the water. Bring the beans back to the pot, add the vegetable broth, and simmer for 60 minutes.

2  In a frying pan, add the olive oil and sauté the onion, garlic, aji, and tomato paste. Once everything is soft and lightly browned, pour it into the beans and mix well. Cover and simmer for another 5 to 10 minutes or until the beans are soft. Add the salt and pepper.

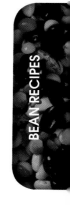

**BEAN RECIPES**

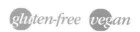 *gluten-free* *vegan*

**Per Serving:** Kcal 318, Protein 16g, Carb 50g, Fat 6g, Sodium 311mg, Dietary Fiber 17g

**Daily Values:** Fiber 68%, Vit C 3%, Vit A 14%, Vit D 0%, Calcium 2%, Iron 2%

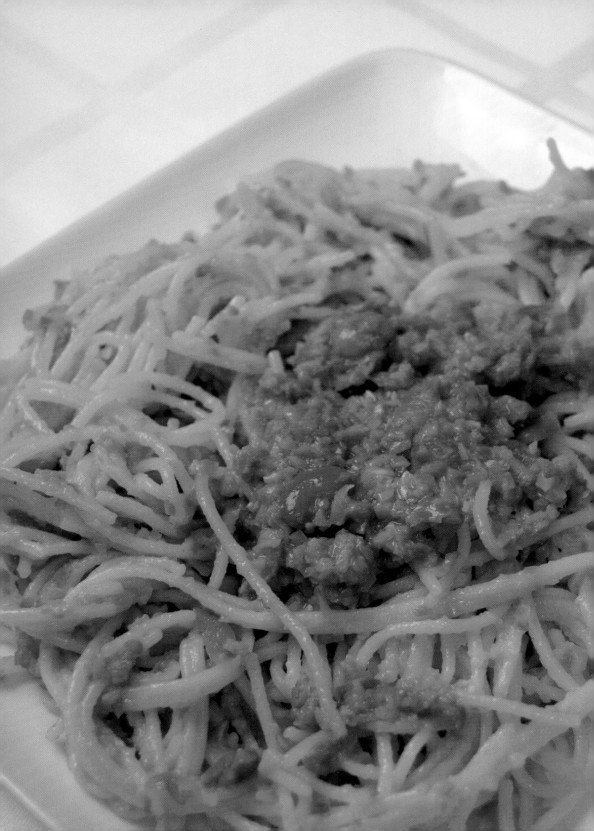

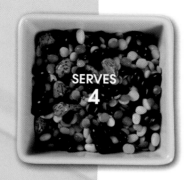

# FAVA PESTO

*This recipe was specially created for this project by Jason D'Angelo of San Francisco's Water- bar. We love the flavor of fava beans, and this preparation lets them shine with the bright citrus notes of orange zest. We served it over quinoa pasta for a healthy, gluten-free entrée.*

## Ingredients

3 cups fava beans, shelled from their pods and peels
Zest of 1 large orange
1 large orange, juiced
4 tablespoons olive oil
Salt to taste

## Directions

1. In a medium saucepan, bring salted water to a rolling boil and blanch the fava beans for no longer than 1 minute. Immediately drain the beans and peel the skins while hot. Discard the skins and keep the beans.

2. Combine all of the ingredients in a food processor and lightly pulse until smooth and evenly combined. Add more salt to taste if you desire. You can refrigerate the pesto in an airtight container for up to 2 days if you top it with a light layer of oil.

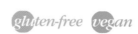

*gluten-free* *vegan*

Per Serving: Kcal 271, Protein 10g, Carb 28g, Fat 14g, Sodium 301mg, Dietary Fiber 7g
Daily Values: Fiber 29%, Vit C 25%, Vit A 1%, Vit D 0%, Calcium 5%, Iron 11%

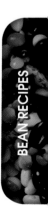

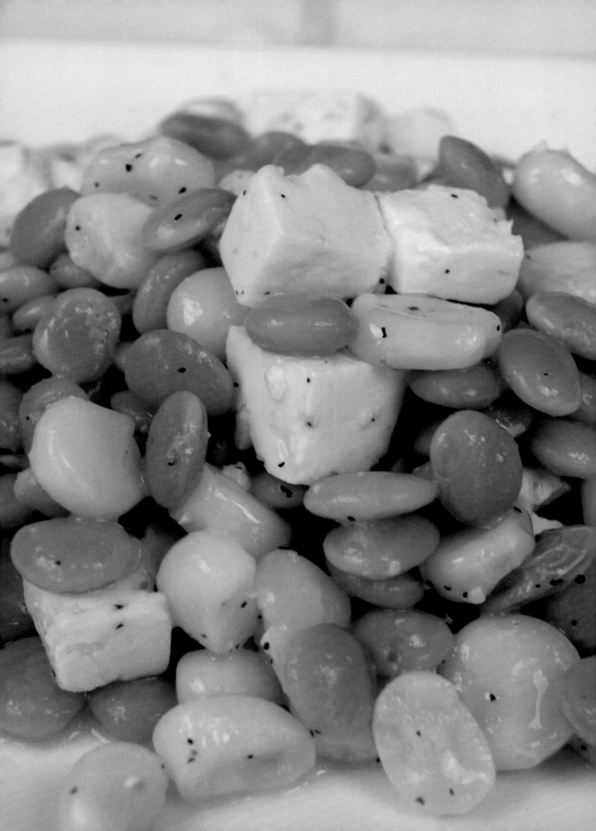

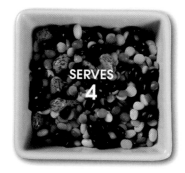

SERVES
4

# LIMA BEANS WITH CHOCLO AND FETA

*Choclo is a Peruvian word for a specific kind of corn with extra large kernels. These days, you can find frozen choclo in Latino markets, and we really recommend you seek it out. The large kernels have a unique sweetness and a wonderful texture. Choclo, paired with lima beans and feta, is a wonderful mélange of sweet and savory. If you can't find choclo, you can use yellow or white corn, preferably fresh, though frozen will do. This dish makes a savory side dish or a wonderful main course for vegetarians.*

## Ingredients

2 cups fresh or frozen choclo (corn)
2 cups fresh or frozen lima beans
8 ounces feta cheese, cubed
2 tablespoons olive oil
3 tablespoons lime juice
1 tablespoon aji
Salt and pepper to taste

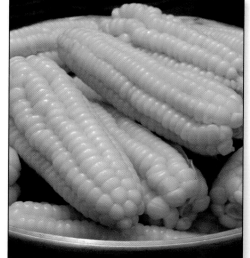

## Directions

1. Mix all of the ingredients (except the salt and pepper) in a bowl and combine well. Season with salt and pepper.

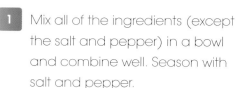
gluten-free  powerstar  vegetarian

**Per Serving:** Kcal 388, Protein 16g, Carb 39g, Fat 20g, Sodium 657mg, Dietary Fiber 7g
**Daily Values:** Fiber 26%, Vit C 25%, Vit A 13%, Vit D 0%, Calcium 31%, Iron 16%

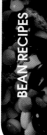
BEAN RECIPES

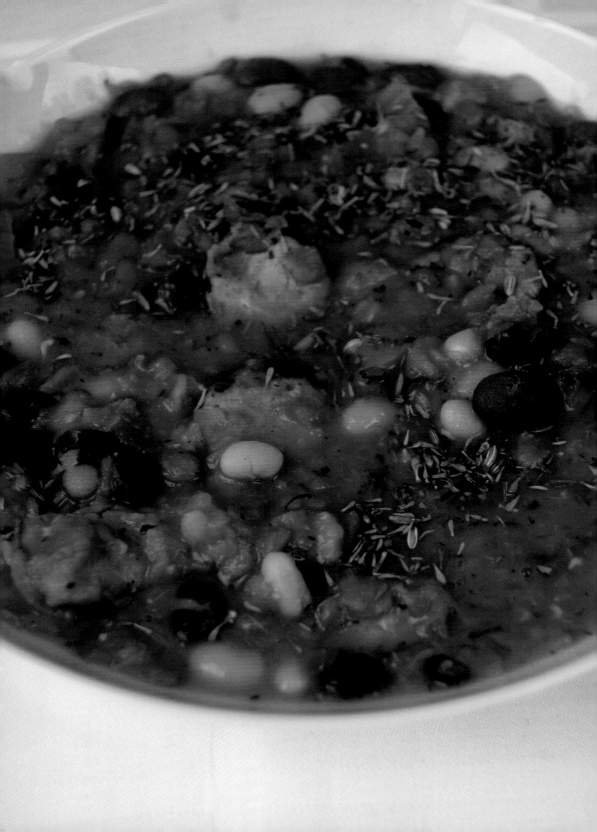

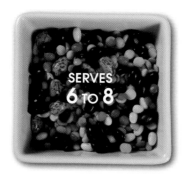

SERVES
6 to 8

# CHICKEN SAUSAGE MIXED BEAN SOUP

*This is a hearty and satisfying soup that's just perfect on a fall evening. You'll get plenty of protein and flavor, yet the chicken sausage is a nice option for low-fat meat.*

## Ingredients

2 cups dried mixed beans

32 ounces chicken broth

1 cup sliced carrots

1 cup sliced celery

1 tablespoon olive oil

1 medium onion, chopped

1 teaspoon garlic, crushed

4 links chicken sausage, sliced

1 tablespoon Herbes de Provence

Salt and pepper to taste

## Directions

**1** Soak the beans for four hours, then discard the water. Place the beans in a pot with enough water to cover them and bring to a boil. Boil for about 1 minute, uncovered. Drain the beans and discard the water.

**2** Bring the beans back to the pot, add the chicken broth, and simmer for 30 minutes. Add the carrots and celery. Continue simmering, uncovered.

**3** Add the olive oil to a frying pan and sauté the onion with garlic, chicken sausage, and herbs. Once everything is soft and lightly browned, pour it into the bean soup. If it seems the soup is getting too thick, add another cup of broth. Cover the beans and simmer for another 30 minutes or until beans are soft. Season with salt and pepper.

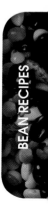

BEAN RECIPES

*gluten-free*

**Per Serving:** Kcal 317, Protein 24g, Carb 40g, Fat 7g, Sodium 342mg, Dietary Fiber 11g

**Daily Values:** Fiber 44%, Vit C 7%, Vit A 64%, Vit D 0%, Calcium 12%, Iron 27%

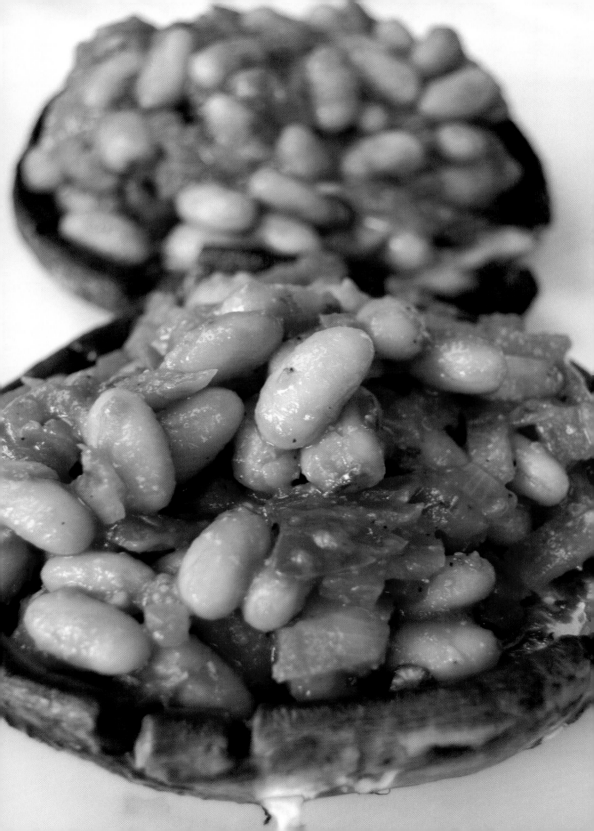

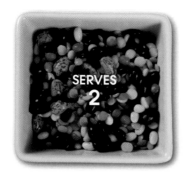

# WHITE BEAN–STUFFED PORTABELLAS

*Portabellas have a wonderful meaty flavor that can satisfy vegetarians and omnivores alike. Add the beans, garlic, and tomato, and this becomes an Italian-inspired entrée.*

## Ingredients

½ cup chopped red onion

1 tablespoon minced garlic

1 tablespoon olive oil

½ cup tomato sauce

1 (15-ounce) can cannellini beans, drained and rinsed

1 tablespoon dried oregano

2 large portabella caps, cleaned

Olive oil spray

salt and pepper to taste

## Directions

1. In a medium saucepan, sauté the onion and garlic in olive oil over high heat until the onion is translucent, roughly 1 to 2 minutes. Add the tomato sauce and stir the mixture. Add the cannellini beans, oregano, and the salt and pepper to taste. Cook for 5 minutes over medium heat. Remove from the heat and set aside.

2. Fry each portabella mushroom cap on each side for about 5 minutes in a hot pan prepared with olive oil spray.

3. Remove from the heat and stuff the caps with the filling.

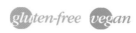 *gluten-free* *vegan*

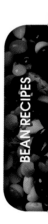

BEAN RECIPES

**Per Serving:** Kcal 283, Protein 15g, Carb 43g, Fat 8g, Sodium 334mg, Dietary Fiber 11g
**Daily Values:** Fiber 44%, Vit C 16%, Vit A 7%, Vit D 0%, Calcium 17%, Iron 36%

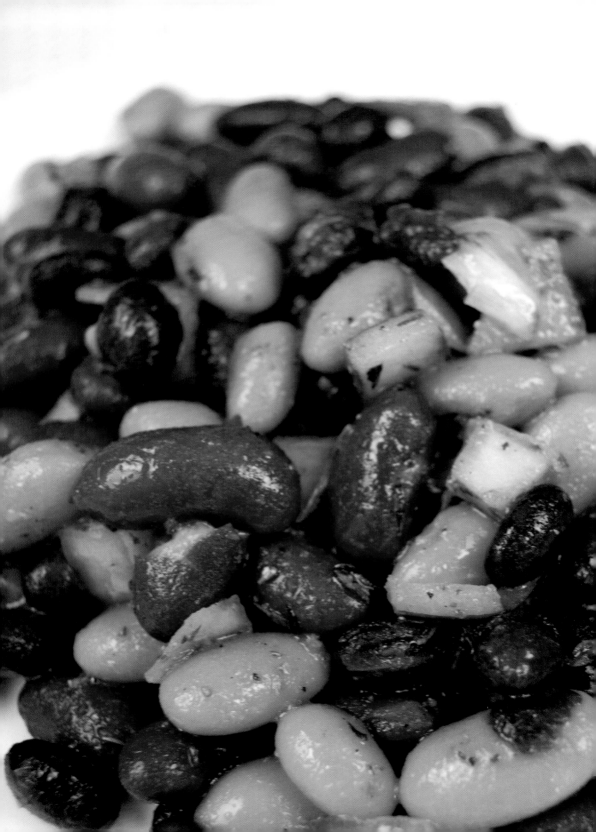

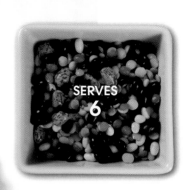

# THREE BEAN SALAD

*This is an Americana classic that still stands up as a summer staple. It's a great alternative side to potato salad and cole slaw at barbeques and picnics.*

## Ingredients

1 (15-ounce) can black beans, drained and rinsed
1 (15-ounce) can kidney beans, drained and rinsed
1 (15-ounce) can canary beans, drained and rinsed
1 red onion, diced
2 tablespoons olive oil
2 tablespoons red wine vinegar
½ teaspoon garlic powder
1 teaspoon dried basil
1 teaspoon dried thyme
1 teaspoon dried oregano
Salt and pepper to taste

## Directions

1. Combine all of the ingredients in a large bowl and gently fold together until evenly incorporated. Chill for at least one hour to let the flavors release and combine.

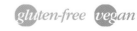

**Per Serving:** Kcal 368, Protein 17g, Carb 60g, Fat 6g, Sodium 52mg, Dietary Fiber 12g
**Daily Values:** Fiber 49%, Vit C 4%, Vit A 0%, Vit D 0%, Calcium 5%, Iron 18%

BEAN RECIPES

# 13 ⌒ PURPLE POTATOES

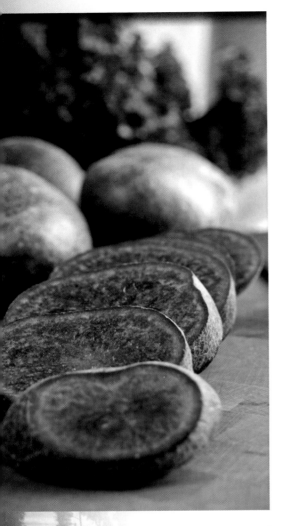

## OVERVIEW

**PURPLE POTATOES ARE** relatively new to the United States, but they've been a staple of the Peruvian diet since the time of the Incas, when they were reserved for kings. While there are several varieties of the purple potato, we most commonly see small spuds, about the size of a walnut. They can, however, grow to much larger sizes and more oblong shapes.

The difference between purple potatoes and yellow varieties is, of course, their color, but also the health benefits associated with that color. These heirloom fingerlings are packed full of anthocyanin, a pigment that acts as an antioxidant. Much of the pigmentation is found in the potato skins, so it's important to cook them with the skin on for maximum health benefits.

Potatoes are a remarkably diverse and nutritious New World food—in Peru there are over 3,000 kinds! When visiting the local open markets, you'll discover countless potato varieties in an array of colors and shapes.

Potatoes are generally a very versatile food and the purple variety is no different. Their pigment offers added nutritional benefits and their color brings interest to more traditional dishes, livening up vegetable roasts, stews, or even a salade Niçoise.

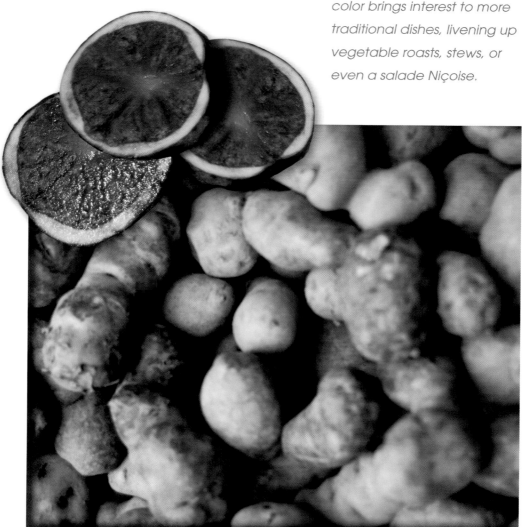

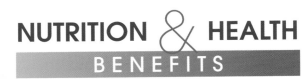

# NUTRITION & HEALTH
## BENEFITS

ANTICANCER

BLOOD PRESSURE CONTROL

BRAIN HEALTHY

HEART HEALTHY

HELPS CONTROL DIABETES

HELPS PROTECT LIVER

Purple potatoes offer an array of essential nutrients, including complex carbohydrates, folic acid, potassium, and vitamin C. Purple potatoes are also rich in anthocyanins, the phytochemical responsible for their purple color and their impressive health benefits.

Purple potatoes pack two to three times the antioxidants of yellow or white potatoes, which means more free-radical scavenging.

When you eat purple potatoes, the anthocyanins are absorbed directly into the blood stream, which has a healing effect on the liver and helps to decrease blood pressure.

Anthocyanins can help control blood sugar levels by breaking up glucose.

Because they fight oxidative stressors that can lead to disease, anthocyanins have been linked with cancer prevention and reducing cancer cell growth as well.

Anthocyanins are an anti-aging power food as they support brain health and cognitive functioning.

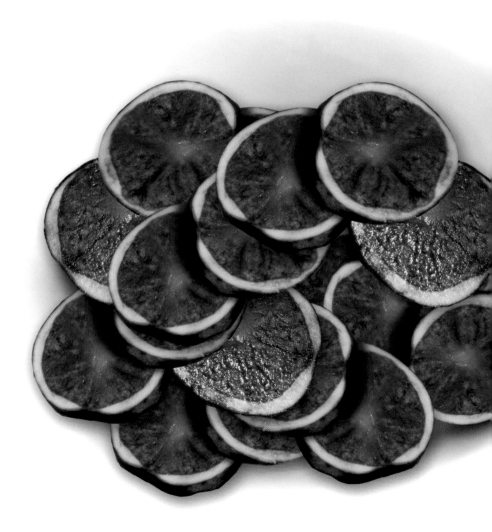

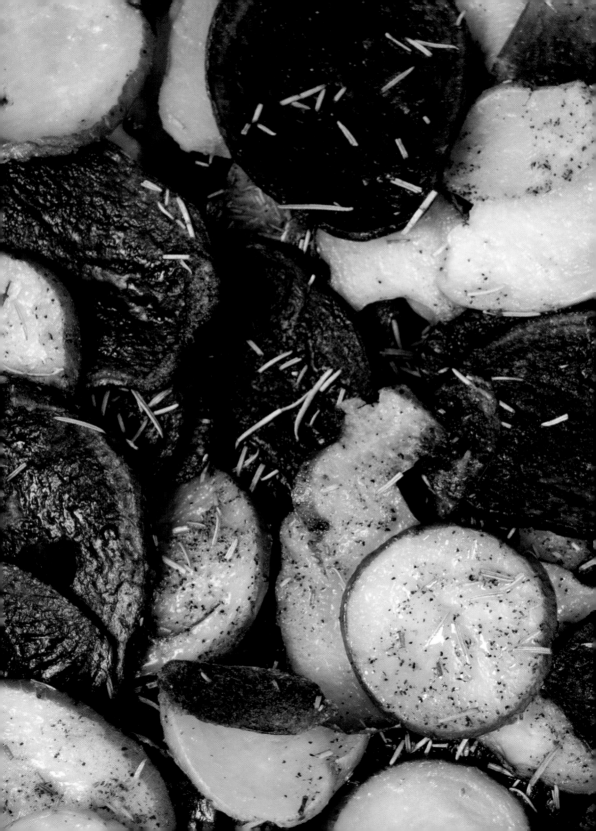

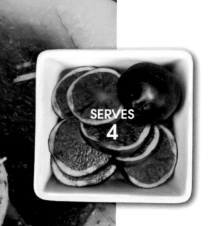

# TRI-COLORED SCALLOPED POTATOES

*This dish uses simple ingredients but delivers impressive results. Once sliced, the thinly layered potatoes in three colors create a beautiful dish with delicate texture.*

**SERVES 4**

## Ingredients

3 medium red potatoes
3 medium yellow potatoes
3 medium purple potatoes
2 tablespoons olive oil
1 sprig rosemary leaves, chopped
Salt and pepper to taste

## Directions

1. Preheat the oven to 400 degrees F. Wash the potatoes and thinly slice with a mandolin or sharp knife. Lightly coat a 9-inch baking dish with nonstick spray.

2. Layer the potatoes in the baking dish, mixing the colors together. Drizzle with olive oil and season with the rosemary and salt and pepper.

3. Cover with foil and bake for 30 minutes. Remove the foil and bake an additional 5 to 10 minutes, or until golden brown.

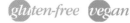 

Per Serving: Kcal 397, Protein 8g, Carb 76g, Fat 7g, Sodium 28mg, Dietary Fiber 5g
Daily Values: Fiber 18%, Vit C 63%, Vit A 0%, Vit D 0%, Calcium 3%, Iron 20%

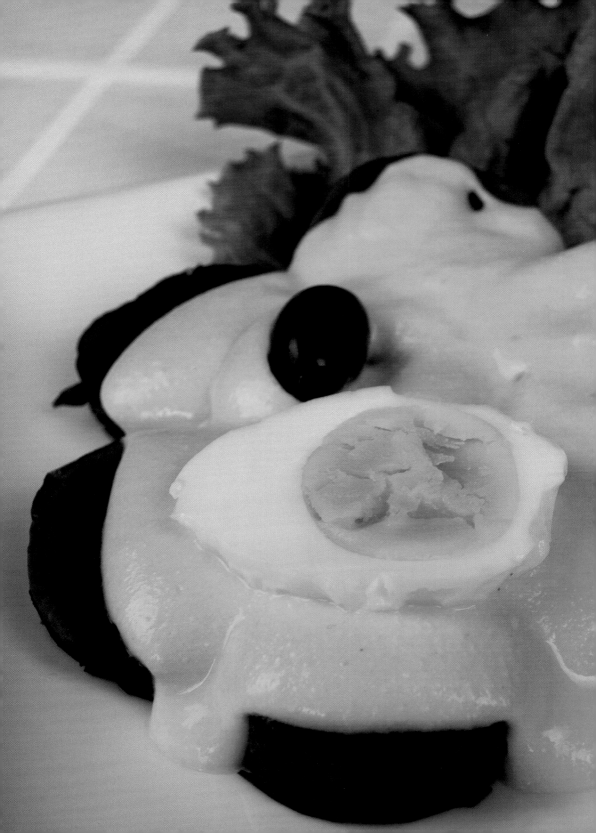

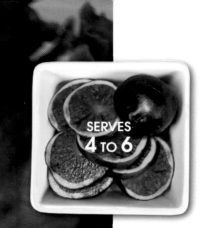

# PURPLE POTATOES
# A LA HUANCAINA

*This is another traditional Peruvian dish, featuring huancaina, a very popular sauce with a mild, tasty flavor. The pairing of potatoes and creamy cheese sauce makes an instant comfort classic.*

## Ingredients

¼ to ½ cup aji sauce (based on your preference for hot/spicy)
10 ounces queso fresco
½ to 1 cup milk
1 ounce or 8 soda crackers
1 pound purple potatoes, boiled and sliced

### For garnish:
2 hard-boiled eggs
10 olives
Lettuce leaves

## Directions

**1** In a blender, combine the aji, cheese, ½ the milk, and soda crackers. Blend until it reaches a medium consistency, adding more milk as needed.

**2** Prepare a plate with the sliced potatoes, cover with the huancaina sauce, and garnish with eggs, olives, and lettuce.

 *vegetarian*

Per Serving: Kcal 213, Protein 10g, Carb 25g, Fat 7g, Sodium 184mg, Dietary Fiber 1g
Daily Values: Fiber 5%, Vit C 0%, Vit A 7%, Vit D 5%, Calcium 21%, Iron 3%

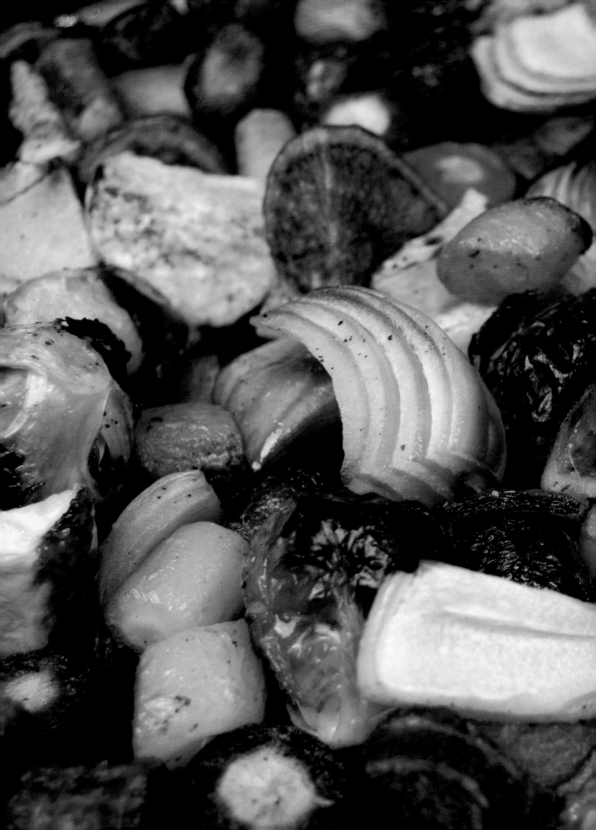

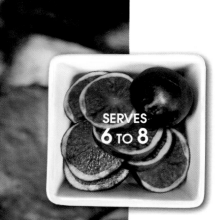

SERVES
6 TO 8

# ROASTED PURPLE POTATOES AND RED ONION

*Sometimes the simplest dishes are the best, and roasted vegetables provide pure, comforting flavor that's hard to beat. Here, we used purple potatoes and red onions as a base recipe, but you can also add cubed butternut squash, parsnips, or yellow potatoes for a more colorful mélange.*

## Ingredients

10 purple potatoes, cubed
2 medium red onions, cubed
2 cups of vegetables in season, cubed
4 cloves garlic, crushed
3 sprigs rosemary, finely chopped
4 tablespoons olive oil
Salt and pepper to taste

## Directions

1   Preheat the oven to 450 degrees F. In a large bowl, toss the vegetables, garlic, and rosemary in the olive oil and mix to coat. Spread the mixture evenly in a roasting pan. Season with salt and pepper.

2   Place in the oven and roast for roughly 20 minutes or until golden brown and thoroughly cooked.

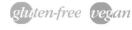

*gluten-free* *vegan*

Per Serving: Kcal 291, Protein 6g, Carb 49g, Fat 8g, Sodium 36mg, Dietary Fiber 5g
Daily Values: Fiber 20%, Vit C 11%, Vit A 42%, Vit D 0%, Calcium 2%, Iron 3%   Purple Potatoes ⌒ 209

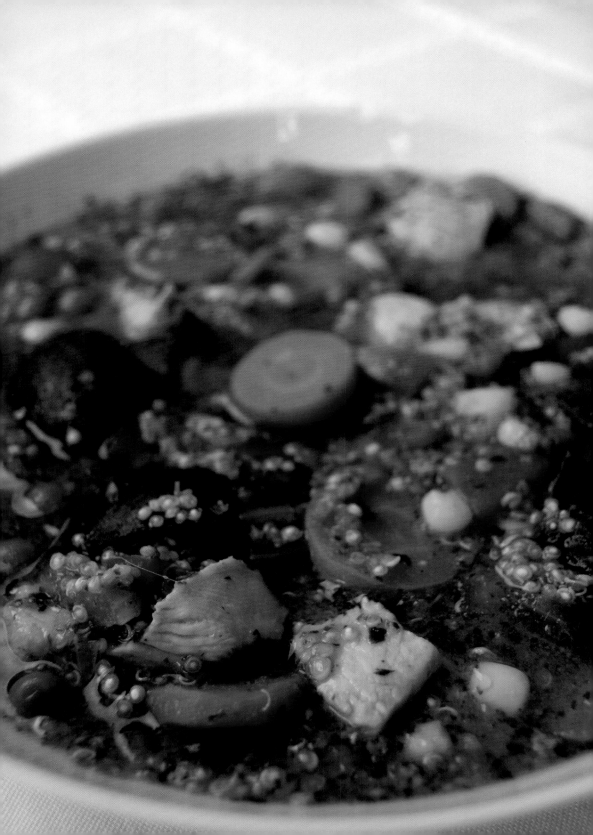

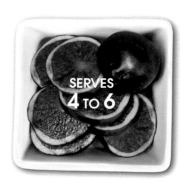

# PURPLE POTATO CILANTRO SOUP

*This hearty soup is a power-food powerhouse. Loaded with nutrients from cilantro, purple potatoes, and quinoa, this soup is both colorful and flavorful.*

SERVES 4 TO 6

## Ingredients

1 bunch cilantro leaves

32 ounces chicken broth

1 tablespoon olive oil

1 medium onion, chopped

5 cloves garlic, chopped

1 pound chicken breast,
   cut into bite-sized pieces

3 celery sticks, chopped

3 medium purple potatoes, diced

2 carrots, sliced

1 cup dry/raw quinoa

½ red bell pepper, chopped

½ cup frozen peas (or fresh if possible)

½ cup frozen corn (or fresh if possible)

## Directions

1. In a blender, liquefy the cilantro with the broth. Put all 32 ounces of the broth into the blender with cilantro. Set aside.

2. Sauté the onion and the garlic until soft and translucent. Add the chicken breast pieces and mix well.

3. In a large stock pot, combine the sautéed mixture with the celery, liquefied cilantro broth, purple potatoes, and carrots. Bring to a boil.

4. Add the quinoa and the bell pepper.

5. Once the quinoa is cooked, about 10 to 15 minutes, add the peas and the corn. Heat until thoroughly warmed.

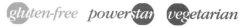

*gluten-free powerstar vegetarian*

**Per Serving:** Kcal 348, Protein 27g, Carb 47g, Fat 5g, Sodium 358mg, Dietary Fiber 7g
**Daily Values:** Fiber 29%, Vit C 59%, Vit A 188%, Vit D 0%, Calcium 7%, Iron 16%

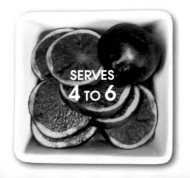

# AJI DE GALLINA OVER PURPLE POTATOES

*Aji de gallina is a beloved traditional Peruvian chicken dish with a consistency somewhere between a hearty stew and a creamy risotto. You can serve it with quinoa, rice, or any other grain, but we like it over purple potatoes for added color and health benefits.*

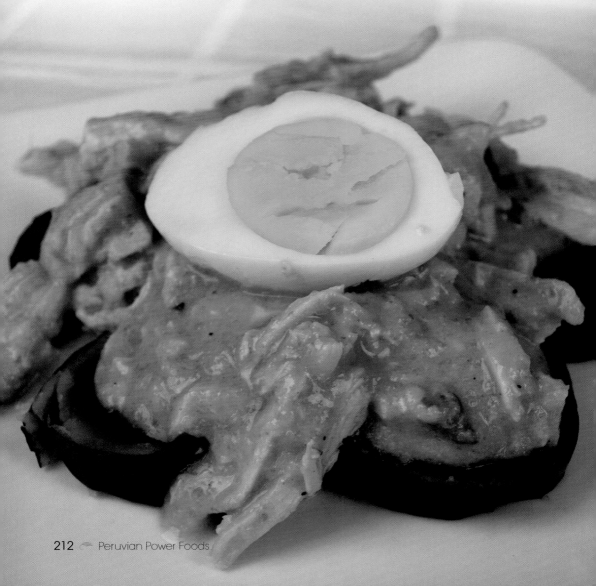

## Ingredients

3 slices whole grain bread
1 cup chicken broth
1 tablespoon olive oil
5 garlic cloves, sliced
1 medium white onion, chopped
1 tablespoon cumin
2 tablespoons aji paste
2 teaspoons each, salt and pepper

16 ounces cooked chicken
   breast, shredded
1 cup evaporated milk
2 ounces walnuts, cut into pieces
2 ounces shredded Parmesan cheese
2 hard-boiled eggs, sliced
10 purple potatoes (boiled for 20
   minutes until tender and sliced)

## Directions

1  Shred the bread into small pieces and place it in the chicken broth to soak. Set aside.

2  Sauté the garlic and onion in the oil until tender and translucent. Add the cumin, aji, and salt and pepper to the pan. This blend is called *aderezo*. Add the *aderezo* to the soaking bread. Blend the mixture with a handheld mixer or a blender until pureed.

3  Pour the pureed sauce into a sauce pan over low heat. Add the shredded chicken and the evaporated milk. Simmer for 5 to 10 minutes, stirring constantly to prevent burning at bottom. Stir in the walnuts and cheese. Serve on top of the purple potatoes and garnish with hard-boiled eggs.

**Per Serving:** Kcal 560, Protein 42g, Carb 62g, Fat 16g, Sodium 513mg, Dietary Fiber 5g
**Daily Values:** Fiber 22%, Vit C 6%, Vit A 6%, Vit D 11%, Calcium 34%, Iron 17%

# 14 ⌒ CILANTRO

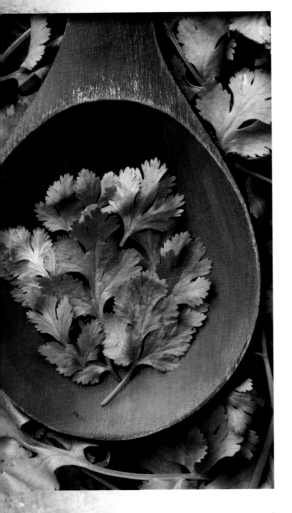

## OVERVIEW

**DRAWN FROM THE CORIANDER** plant, cilantro is a leafy green herb that bears a resemblance to Italian or flat-leaf parsley. Hasty shoppers often confuse the two, but one sniff will immediately distinguish them.

Cilantro has a bold flavor that falls under the "love it or hate it" category. And in this case, that's for good scientific reason. A percentage of people can't taste all its flavor compounds, and for that group, the taste is metallic or soapy. For others though, cilantro has a bright, pleasing flavor that livens up any dish.

While cilantro isn't one of the primary herbs we use in the States, you'll see that every Peruvian keeps fresh cilantro in the refrigerator. Besides being a flavorful garnish and dish topper, it is often the centerpiece of sauces, dips, soups, and stews.

Long popular in Mexican, Indian, and South American cuisine, cilantro is relatively new to us in North America. With antioxidant, antifungal, and antibacterial properties, this is one powerful herb. It also supports heart health and anti-diabetic activity, so if you're one that appreciates this bold flavor, make cilantro a regular part of your diet as it's one of the hardest-working herbs when it comes to your health.

*In Peruvian cuisine, cilantro is often used as the base for a dish, while the rest of the ingredients are built around its unique flavor. The most common of these dishes is seco, a traditional beef stew. We've included our own recipe for seco here, as this is one authentic dish not to be missed.*

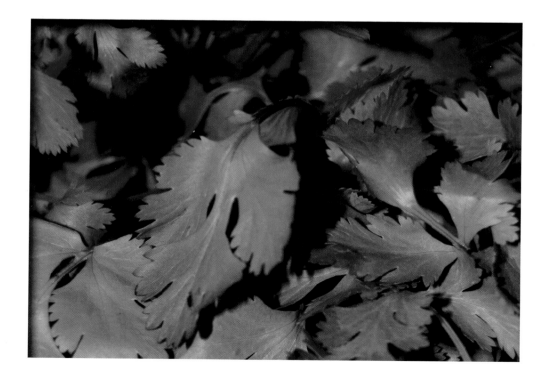

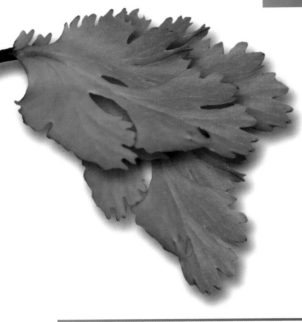

# NUTRITION & HEALTH

ANTIBACTERIAL

ANTIFUNGAL

ANTIOXIDANT

DIABETES FRIENDLY

HEART HEALTHY

PHYTONUTRIENT DENSE

SLEEP AID

Cilantro is rich in beta-carotene; folic acid; niacin; riboflavin; vitamin A; and vitamin C, a natural antioxidant. It's also a good source of calcium, iron, magnesium, manganese, and potassium.

The potassium in cilantro supports cellular health and body fluids that help control heart rate and blood pressure.

Because cilantro is also rich in iron, it supports red blood cell production.

The leaves and stem tips are also rich in numerous antioxidant flavonoids that scavenge free radicals and help prevent the onset of heart disease and cancer.

Studies show that cilantro has a protective effect on the cells of the heart, helping to prevent heart attacks and oxidative damage.

Research proves that both the stems and the leaves of cilantro may be helpful for diabetics.

Some studies suggest that cilantro may improve sleep quality.

Cilantro has also been shown to lower blood sugar.

Cilantro has demonstrated both antibacterial and antifungal properties. In fact, some dental schools are studying how cilantro might be used for oral health.

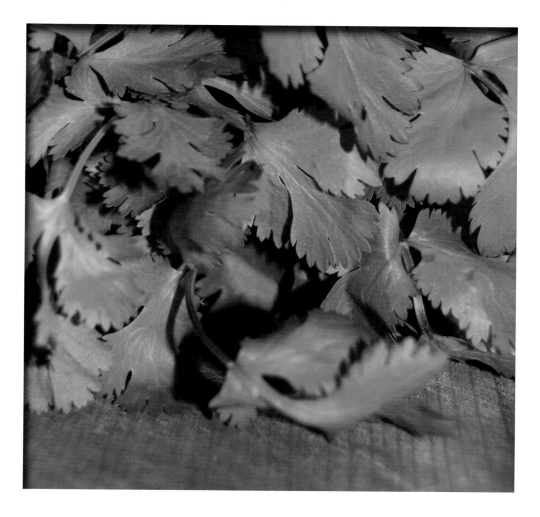

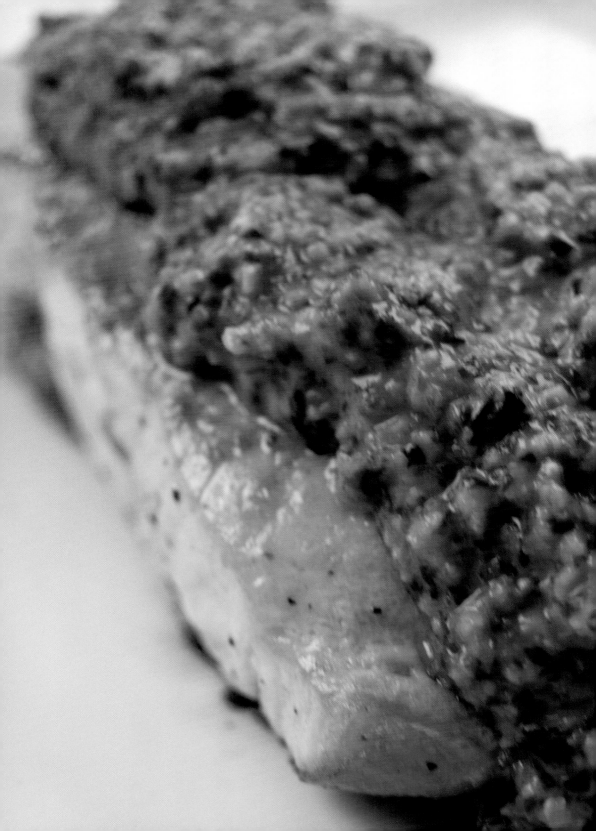

SERVES
4

# CILANTRO PESTO

*This is a fresh and healthful take on a more traditional pesto. With the power of both cilantro and sacha inchi oil and seeds, it's a potent antioxidant blend with extra omega-3s. We especially love this over grilled or poached salmon.*

## Ingredients

1 bunch cilantro
½ cup sacha inchi seeds
2 tablespoons sacha inchi oil
2 tablespoons lime juice
Salt to taste

## Directions

1. Roughly remove the cilantro leaves from the stems.

2. Combine the cilantro leaves, sacha inchi seeds, sacha inchi oil, and lime juice in a food processor and puree until smooth. Season with salt.

**CILANTRO RECIPES**

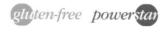

*gluten-free* *powerstar*

**Per Serving:** Kcal 215, Protein 7g, Carb 4g, Fat 18g, Sodium 7mg, Dietary Fiber 2g
**Daily Values:** Fiber 9%, Vit C 8%, Vit A 17%, Vit D 0%, Calcium 3%, Iron 3%

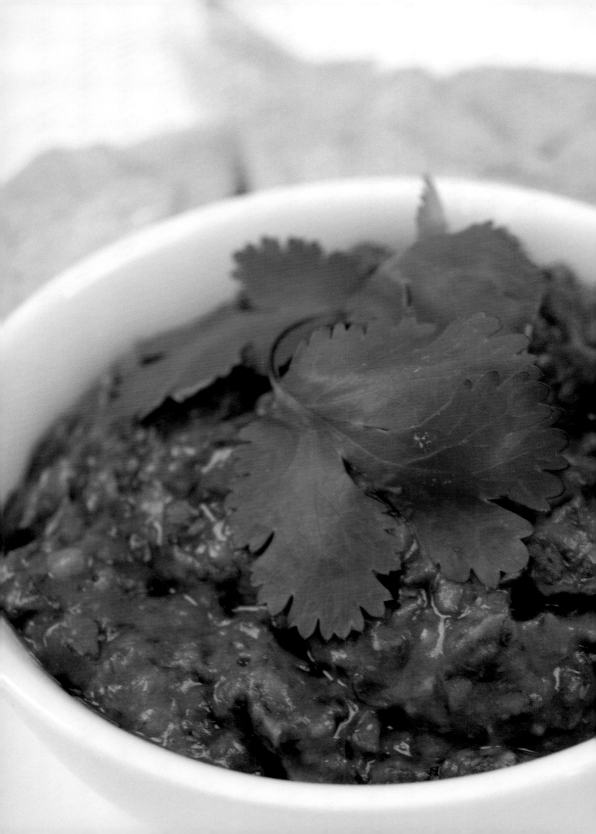

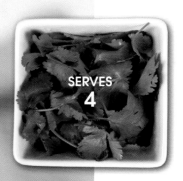

**SERVES 4**

# BLACK BEAN DIP

*This is an easy dip to assemble, and it's the perfect complement to blue corn chips and Amazonian guacamole (see page 91). Top it all off with a yacito cocktail (see page 249).*

(see page 91)

(see page 249)

## Ingredients

1 (16-ounce) can black beans, drained and rinsed
   (reserve the liquid)
1½ tablespoons reserved black bean juice
1 teaspoon lime juice
1 tablespoon sacha inchi oil
1 tablespoon cilantro paste
Salt to taste

## Directions

1 Combine all of the ingredients in a food processor and blend until smooth.

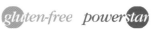

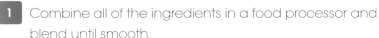

*gluten-free* **powerstar** *vegan*

**Per Serving:** Kcal 183, Protein 10g, Carb 27g, Fat 4g, Sodium 1mg, Dietary Fiber 10g
**Daily Values:** Fiber 40%, Vit C 1%, Vit A 0%, Vit D 0%, Calcium 3%, Iron 13%

SERVES
10

# CILANTRO SECO BEEF STEW

*Seco is one of the most common and beloved dishes in Peru. The flavor of cilantro is the star here, and the cubed beef makes a hearty, satisfying stew that you'll want to add to your regular repertoire.*

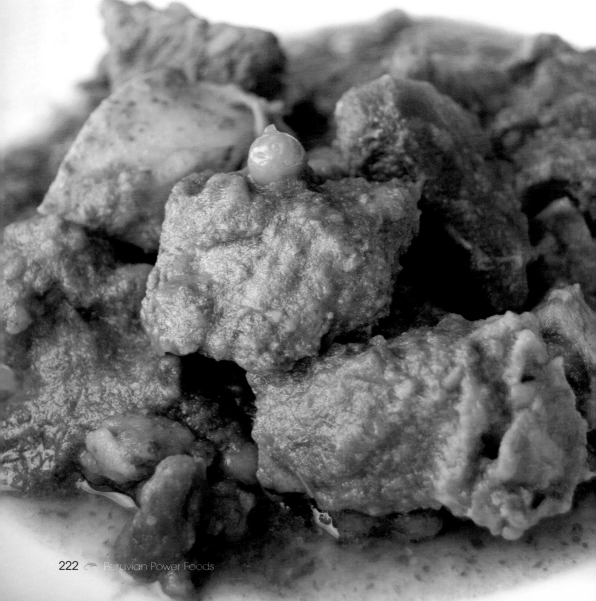

## Ingredients

1 tablespoon olive oil

½ medium onion, chopped

2 garlic cloves, minced

1½ pounds raw beef stewing
   meat (very lean)

1 teaspoon ground cumin

2 cups canned beef broth

1 bunch cilantro, chopped

3 to 4 small unpeeled red potatoes,
   cubed

½ cup frozen carrots

1 cup frozen green peas

## Directions

1. Put 2 teaspoons of the olive oil into a pan and sauté the onions and garlic over medium-high heat.

2. Put the remaining olive oil in a separate pan and sear the beef. Reserve the beef juice. Add the beef and cumin to the onion and garlic mixture. Stir and cook on low heat until the meat is browned on the outside and just cooked through (approximately 5 to 10 minutes, depending on the cube thickness), and then cover.

3. Meanwhile, put the beef broth and cilantro into a blender and blend. Add to the beef mixture. Cover the pan and simmer on low heat for 30 to 40 minutes.

4. Add the potatoes to the pan and cook uncovered for 30 minutes.

5. Add the carrots and peas and cook uncovered for 10 to 15 minutes.

**NOTE:** *If you're using fresh carrots, add them at the same time you add the potatoes and cook for 30 minutes. In Peruvian culture, this dish is served with rice and Peruvian canary beans (see page 189).*

gluten-free

**Per Serving:** Kcal 158, Protein 17g, Carb 12g, Fat 4g, Sodium 231mg, Dietary Fiber 2g
**Daily Values:** Fiber 7%, Vit C 14%, Vit A 25%, Vit D 0%, Calcium 3%, Iron 12%

Cilantro ⌒ 223

**CILANTRO RECIPES**

**SERVES 6**

# JUANES

Juanes *are a classic Amazonian preparation of tightly packed rice cakes encasing meat, olives, and eggs. The rice is flavored with cilantro, and the whole thing is bundled into a ball, wrapped in a banana leaf (or a tamale casing, if you need a substitution), and cooked in a water bath. When you unwrap the bundle, you're left with a perfectly formed rice ball stuffed with delicious, savory filling. These are fun to make and impressive to serve, especially if you leave the chicken bone protruding for dramatic effect.*

## Ingredients

1 onion, chopped

2 cloves garlic

¼ teaspoon cumin

Salt and pepper to taste

1 cup finely chopped cilantro

6 chicken legs

3½ cups water

3 cups rice

2 tablespoons vegetable oil

2 raw eggs

5 hard-boiled eggs

12 olives

12 banana leaves (you can find these in Latino or some Asian markets)

6 lengths of cooking twine, 4 inches long

## Directions

1. Sauté the onion, garlic, cumin, and salt and pepper in hot oil for about 2 minutes. Add the cilantro and mix well. Add the chicken legs and ½ cup water to the sauté pan and cook about 10 minutes, covered.

2. Remove the chicken legs and set aside. To the cilantro mix, add the rice and 3 cups of water, and continue to cook for 12 minutes. Please note: the rice does not need to be cooked all the way through—just started, as you would with arborio rice for risotto.

3. Remove the rice mixture from the heat and add two raw eggs, stirring constantly but gently to avoid cooking the eggs. Let the rice cool about 10 minutes and then separate the rice into 6 equal portions.

4. Lay 2 banana leaves over one another in a cross formation. In the center, place one portion of the previously prepared rice. Place a piece of chicken, 2 halves of the boiled egg, and 2 olives in the center, molding the rice up around the sides as if forming a volcano. Then wrap the banana leaves up and around the mound, tying them together at the top.

5. Repeat step 4 with the ten remaining banana leaves. In a large soup pot, bring salted water to a boil. Add the 6 juanes and let them boil for 25 minutes. Remove them from the pot and leave them to cool. After 30 minutes, unwrap the leaves to reveal the juanes rice balls. Remove them from the banana leaves to plate.

**Per Serving:** Kcal 556, Protein 40g, Carb 24g, Fat 32g, Sodium 279mg, Dietary Fiber 1g
**Daily Values:** Fiber 5%, Vit C 11%, Vit A 15%, Vit D 8%, Calcium 8%, Iron 23%

# 15 ⌒ PAPAYA

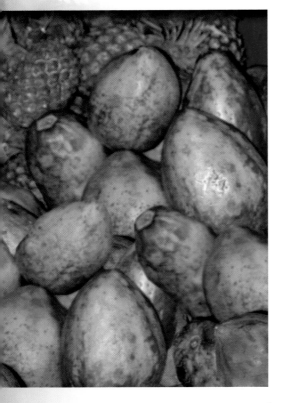

Papaya is ubiquitous in Peru, from the coast to the mountains to the jungle. We ate it for breakfast most mornings when we visited the country, with cool *queso fresco*, sweet bread, and strong coffee. It's also a staple ingredient in the *jugerias*, or juice stands, on every corner. Walk through any open market in Peru, and you'll see counters lined with blenders whipping up fresh papaya, mango, and pineapple.

## OVERVIEW

**THE PAPAYA IS A** tropical fruit that varies between the size of a large mango and a butternut squash. Encased in green skin, the orange flesh is sweet and soft enough to be eaten right out of the rind with a spoon.

Legend has it that when Christopher Columbus first landed in South America, the natives offered his men plentiful amounts of food. However, after so many months at sea with little nourishment, they experienced great digestive pains. They were then offered papaya, which brought intestinal relief. Whether this is true or just a parable about papaya's power, this story reveals one of the fruit's most prized healing properties.

Long a staple in Peruvian culture, the papaya is also used by traditional medicine systems around the world to treat many diseases and ailments, particularly those related to the stomach and digestion. The papaya contains a high concentration of powerful enzymes called proteolytic enzymes, which are also found in our stomachs. These hardworking agents help break down large compounds in the diet and ease digestion, alongside fiber.

Interestingly, papaya is also used as an anti-aging treatment in some organic skin-care lines. Applied topically, the enzymes help eat away dead skin cells and promote cellular regeneration.

*As it is a delicious tropical fruit, papaya can be eaten and enjoyed on its own or in fruit salad. It is also delicious added to smoothies, shakes, salsas, sorbets, and salads.*

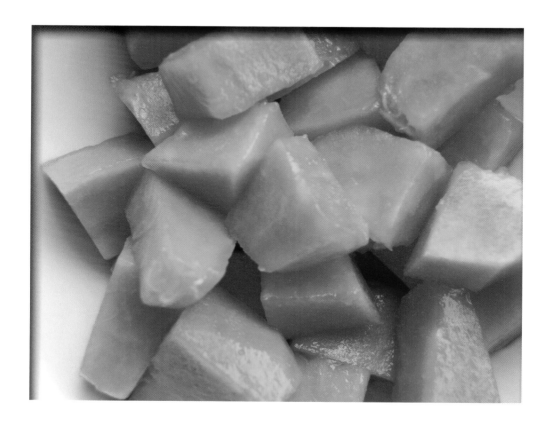

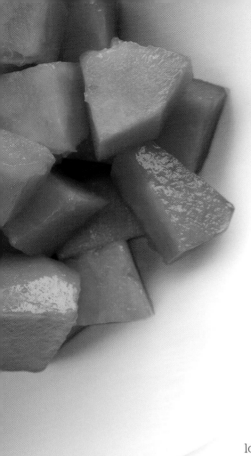

# NUTRITION & HEALTH
## BENEFITS

ANTI-INFLAMMATORY

HEART HEALTHY

SUPPORTS DIGESTIVE HEALTH

SUPPORTS IMMUNE SYSTEM

Rich in vitamin A and vitamin C, papaya is also a good source of fiber, folate, potassium, and vitamin E. It is also a low-calorie fruit loaded with the antioxidant beta-carotene.

Beta-carotene has been linked to a decreased risk of cardiovascular disease and decreased mortality rate from such diseases. Vitamin C has been shown to decrease the risk of cardiovascular disease and heart attacks in women.

Studies have shown that papaya is antibacterial, antifungal, anti-inflammatory, antiviral, hypoglycemic, and neuroprotective.

Oxidative damage to our cells caused by various sources including free radicals may be the root of many signs of aging. So introducing antioxidants, like papaya, that fight free radicals and prevent oxidative damage are a powerful tool in battling the effects of age, both internal and external.

Papaya contains enzymes called proteolytic enzymes, which are commonly found in the human stomach, that help break down large compounds in the diet. These enzymes in combination with the fiber content gives papaya the ability to help with digestive system health.

The fiber in papaya can bind to cancer-causing toxins and flush them away from healthy cells, thus helping to prevent colon cancer. In addition, papaya's beta-carotene, folate, and vitamins C and E are also linked to reduced risk of colon cancer. Those with increased risk of colon cancer should increase their intake of papaya.

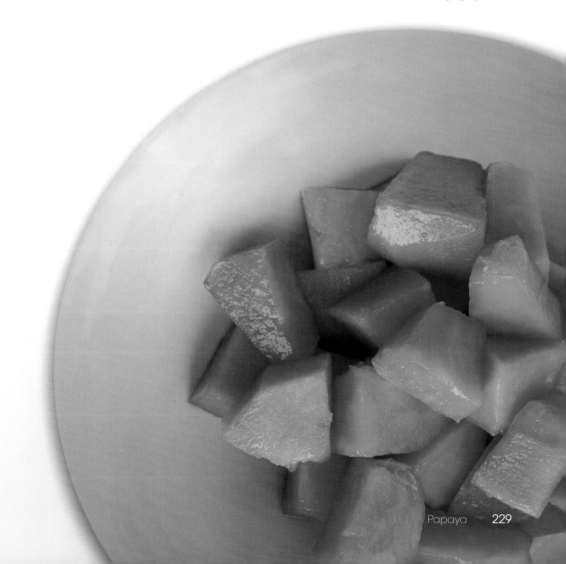

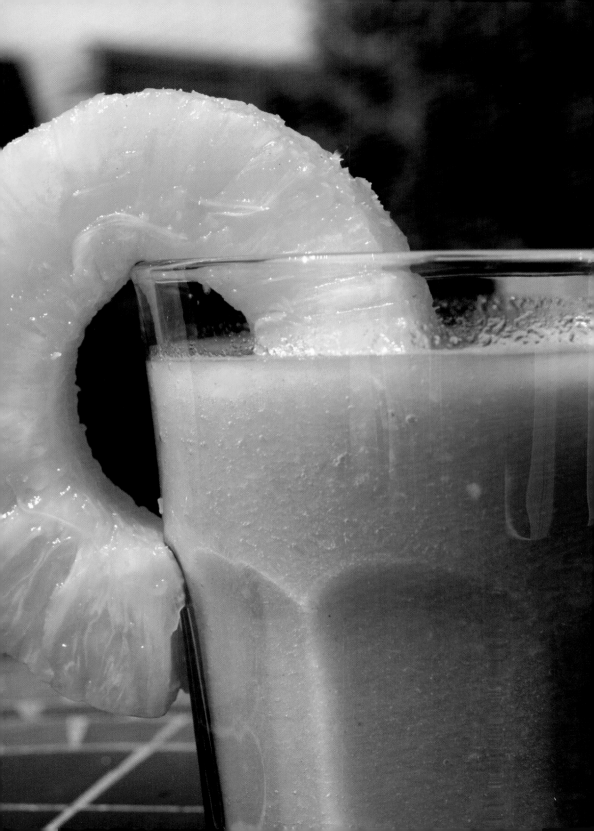

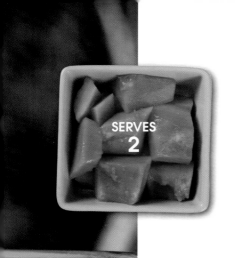

# TROPICAL SMOOTHIE

*There's no better way to transport yourself to the tropics than with a frothy blend of jungle fruit. One taste of this elixir takes us right back to Iquitos, where, each morning, we enjoyed mango and papaya as smooth and sweet as gelato.*

**SERVES 2**

## Ingredients

1 cup chopped mango
1 cup chopped papaya
1 cup chopped pineapple
1½ cups water
1 teaspoon camu camu powder
1 tablespoon yacon

## Directions

1. Combine all of the ingredients in a blender and mix until smooth.

 *gluten-free*  *powerstar*  *vegetarian*

**Per Serving:** Kcal 140, Protein 1g, Carb 39g, Fat 0g, Sodium 16mg, Dietary Fiber 4g
**Daily Values:** Fiber 15%, Vit C 762%, Vit A 30%, Vit D 0%, Calcium 4%, Iron 8%

PAPAYA RECIPES

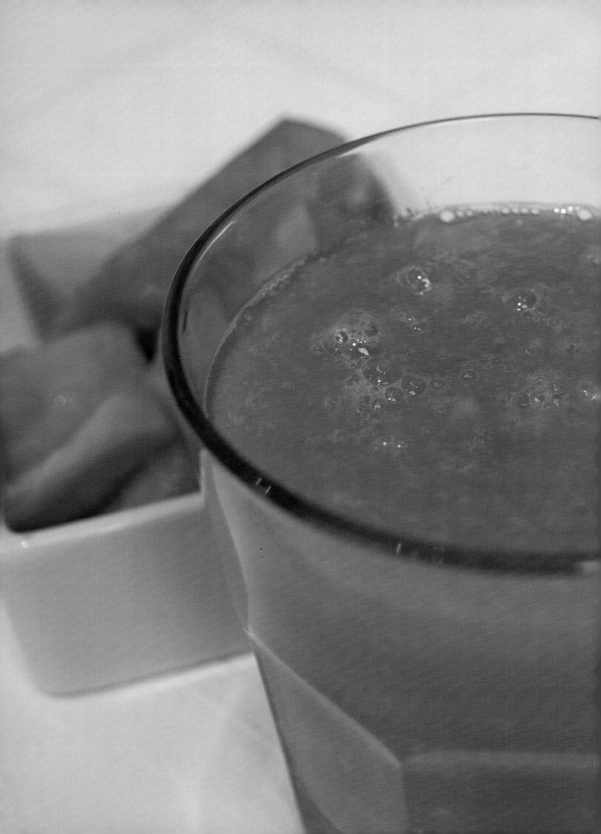

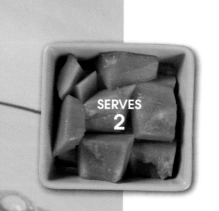

**SERVES
2**

# PAPAYA JUICE

*Maybe you don't have time to do a big juicing production every morning, but if you have papaya on hand, this is the simplest way to enjoy a refreshing, revitalizing juice. It's also good with a spritz of lime if you want to cut the sweetness.*

## Ingredients

2 cups chopped papaya
1 cup water
1 tablespoon agave

## Directions

**1** Combine all of the ingredients in a blender and mix until smooth.

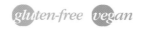 *gluten-free* *vegan*

**Per Serving:** Kcal 86, Protein 1g, Carb 22g, Fat 0g, Sodium 9mg, Dietary Fiber 3g
**Daily Values:** Fiber 10%, Vit C 144%, Vit A 31%, Vit D 0%, Calcium 4%, Iron 1%

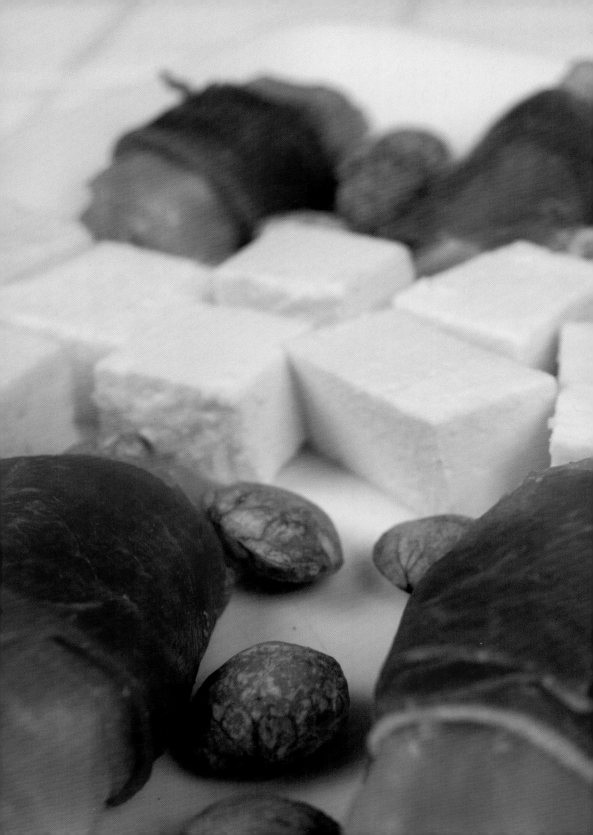

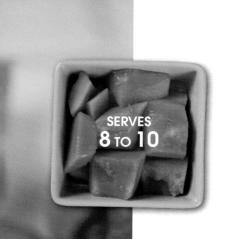

SERVES
**8 TO 10**

# PAPAYA AND PROSCIUTTO

*This is less of a recipe and more of an inspired pairing. We often see cantaloupe wrapped with prosciutto, but why not try the more nutrient-dense and deeply flavored papaya? We served it here with* queso fresco *and* sacha inchi seeds—*a winning combination all around.*

## Ingredients

1 medium papaya
1 package prosciutto, thinly sliced
8 ounces queso fresco, cubed (optional)
20–25 sacha inchi seeds (optional)

## Directions

1. Slice the papaya in half and remove its seeds with a spoon.

2. Cut the papaya into 2 x 1 inch slices. Wrap the individual papaya slices with prosciutto and serve immediately. Sprinkle each slice with queso fresco and sacha inchi seeds, if desired.

PAPAYA RECIPES

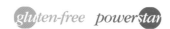

*gluten-free powerstar*

Per Serving: Kcal 88, Protein 7g, Carb 6g, Fat 4g, Sodium 374mg, Dietary Fiber 1g
Daily Values: Fiber 4%, Vit C 48%, Vit A 13%, Vit D 0%, Calcium 8%, Iron 2%

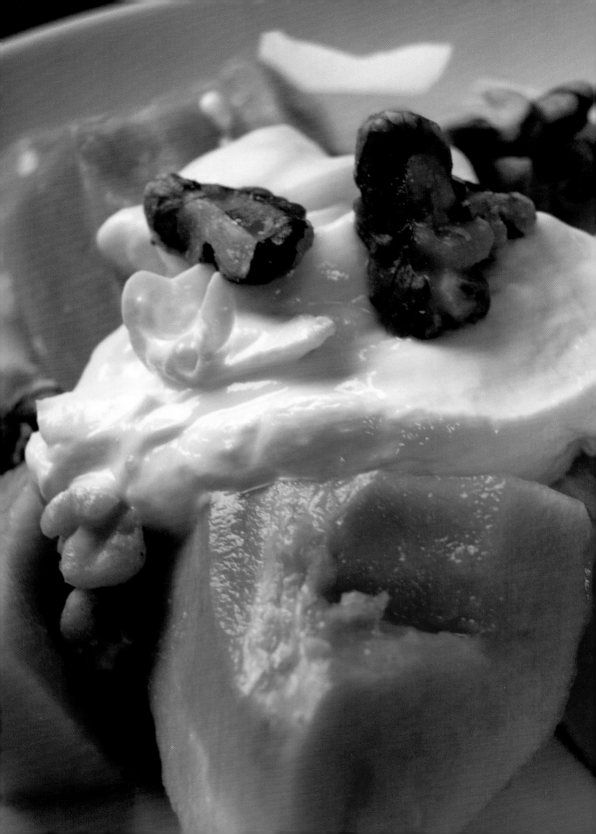

# PAPAYA CUP

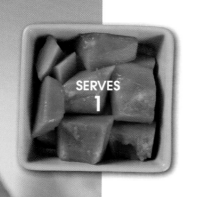

**SERVES 1**

*The natural contours of the papaya, once cleared of its seeds, make a handy serving shape. You can cube the fruit flesh and serve it in a bowl as we've suggested here, or spoon yogurt or cottage cheese right into the center and eat the contents with a spoon.*

## Ingredients

1 cup cubed papaya
½ cup Greek yogurt
1 tablespoon walnut pieces
Honey to drizzle on top (optional)

## Directions

1. Slice the papaya in half and remove its seeds with a spoon. Scoop the flesh from the peel and cube the fruit.

2. Top with Greek yogurt and walnuts. Drizzle with honey if desired.

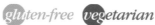

gluten-free  vegetarian

**Per Serving:** Kcal 184, Protein 13g, Carb 25g, Fat 5g, Sodium 48mg, Dietary Fiber 3g
**Daily Values:** Fiber 12%, Vit C 144%, Vit A 31%, Vit D 0%, Calcium 4%, Iron 2%

PAPAYA RECIPES

# 16 ⌒ YACON

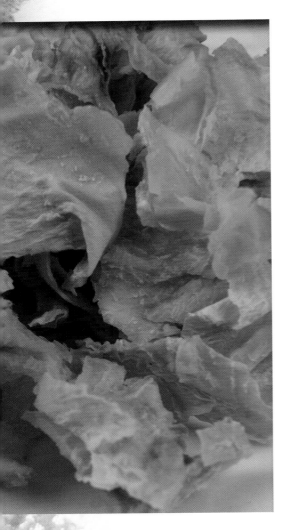

Yacon has a deep, caramelized flavor, approaching the dark sweetness of molasses. Once we discovered all its health benefits, we felt no guilt adding this sweet syrup to all kinds of dishes and desserts.

## OVERVIEW

**A COUSIN OF THE SUNFLOWER,** yacon syrup is processed similarly to maple syrup, though this sweet stuff comes from the root of the yacon plant, a Peruvian tuber similar to the sweet potato. Besides tasting delicious, with a deep, dark caramel flavor, yacon supports intestinal microorganisms with very few calories. Despite its stand-in as a sweetener, for many years in South America it's been used to support digestion and lower blood sugar in those with diabetes. Yacon is naturally low in sugars that elevate blood sugar levels, so it's a perfect low-glycemic sweetener, with a remarkable glycemic index of 1.

In addition to offering a great sweetening alternative to those monitoring blood sugar, yacon is very beneficial for all manner of intestinal health, as it regulates intestinal flora, supports colon health, improves digestion, and promotes the absorption of calcium, the B vitamins, and magnesium. Yacon stimulates the growth of certain probiotics, which can help to relieve constipation. And finally, because of its high antioxidant content, yacon reduces free-radical damage in the body, particularly in the colon.

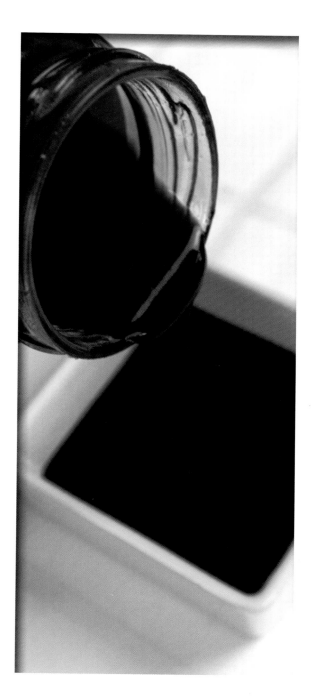

*Yacon can be used in any dish where you might typically choose maple syrup, molasses, or dark agave syrup. It's equally delicious used straight on pancakes or waffles, or baked into breads, stirred into desserts, or drizzled over ice cream.*

# NUTRITION & HEALTH
## BENEFITS

**HELPS CONTROL DIABETES AND
BLOOD SUGAR**

**INCREASES CALCIUM ABSORPTION**

**LOW GLYCEMIC INDEX**

**HELPS PROMOTE WEIGHT LOSS**

Yacon contains probiotics, the good bacteria that occur naturally in our intestines and keep bodily balance in check. Probiotics fight foreign invaders—or bad bacteria—in the gut. And for this reason, probiotics have also been linked to a lowered risk of colon cancer.

Yacon contains nonglycemic carbohydrates, which are a good energy source for diabetics because of their reduced effect on blood sugar levels. Studies also show a reduced glycemic response after people consume yacon, particularly in diabetic individuals.

Combined with soluble fiber, yacon can make you feel fuller while you eat, which can help with weight loss. It slows absorption of sugars into the blood stream.

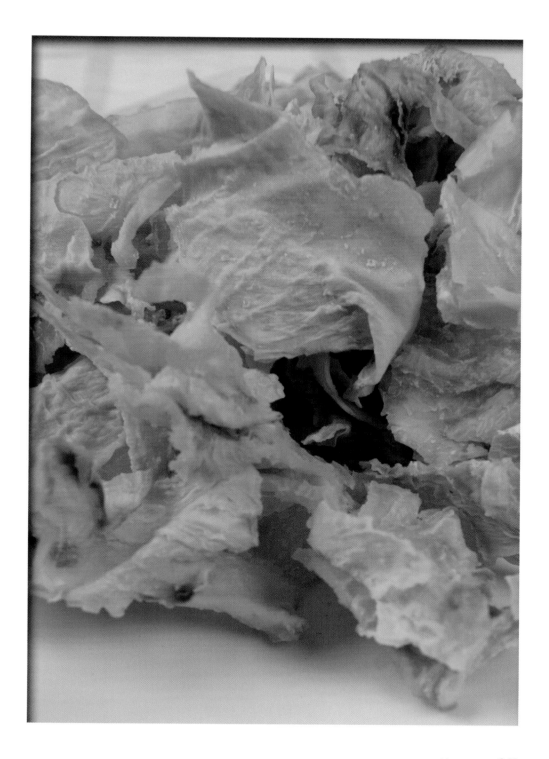

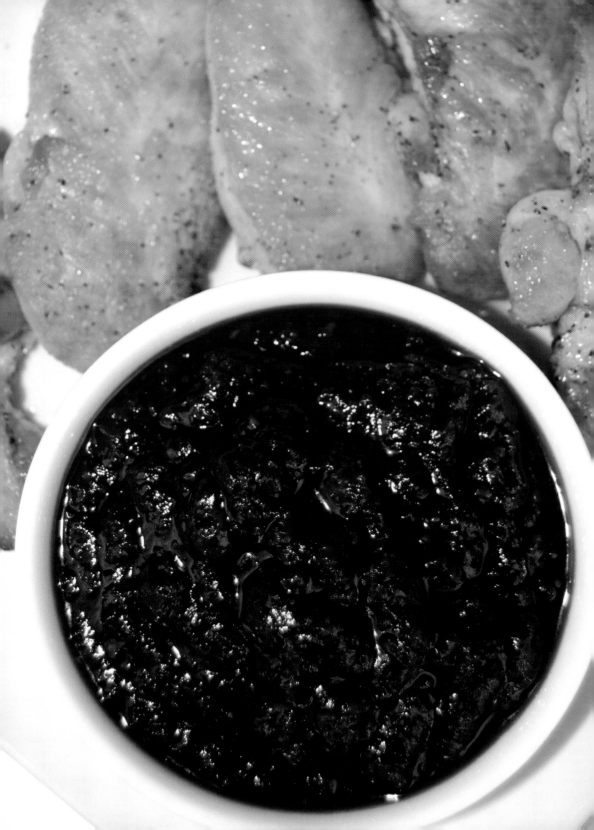

**SERVES
4**

# TANGY BBQ SAUCE

*This recipe was created around yacon's deep flavor by Jason D'Angelo, chef of San Francisco's Waterbar. The sauce is fruity, sweet, and tangy, with just a little kick. Try it on chicken, pork roast, veggies, or summer sausages.*

## Ingredients

1 tablespoon dried cherries

1 tablespoon dried golden raisins

2 heaping tablespoons
   tomato paste

5 tablespoons yacon syrup

1 clove garlic

1 small shallot

¼ jalapeño, chopped

2 tablespoons sherry vinegar

1 tablespoon water

Juice of ½ lime

Salt and pepper to taste

## Directions

**1** In a small saucepan, combine the cherries, raisins, tomato paste, yacon syrup, garlic, shallot, jalapeño, sherry vinegar, and water. Stir to evenly combine ingredients.

**2** Bring the mixture to a boil, reduce the heat to medium, and allow the sauce to simmer and cook down, roughly 20 minutes.

**3** Once the sauce is reduced, use a blender or handheld mixer to blend the sauce to a smooth consistency. Add the lime juice and stir. Season with salt and pepper and enjoy!

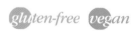

*gluten-free vegan*

**Per Serving:** Kcal 52, Protein 1g, Carb 21g, Fat 0g, Sodium 82mg, Dietary Fiber 1g
**Daily Values:** Fiber 3%, Vit C 8%, Vit A 5%, Vit D 0%, Calcium 1%, Iron 3%

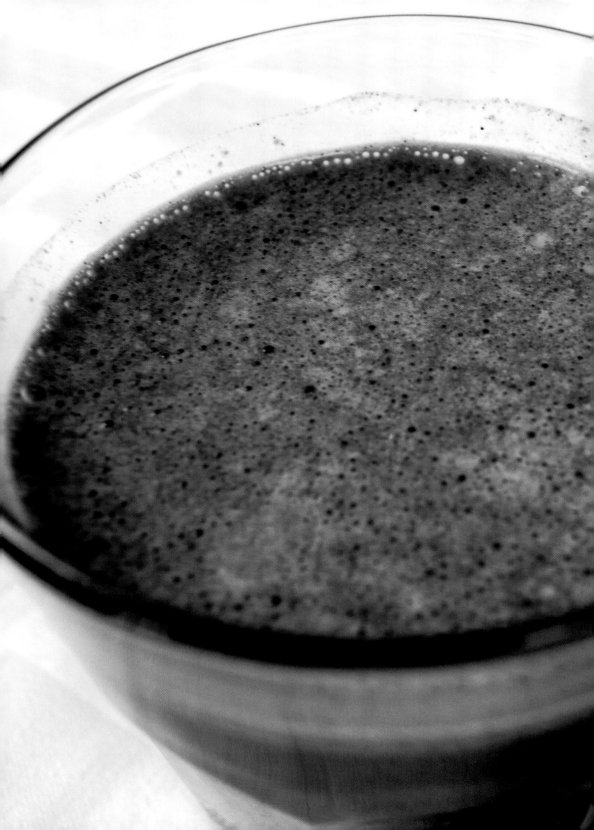

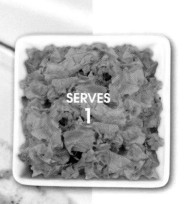

# INCA CHOCOLATE MILK

*It's all the great taste of classic chocolate milk with the power-food boost the Incas enjoyed. Kids will love it too, and they won't even know it's good for them.*

**SERVES 1**

## Ingredients

1 tablespoon maca
1 tablespoon cacao
1 cup milk of your choice (cow, soy, almond, or rice)
1 tablespoon yacon

## Directions

1 Combine all of the ingredients in a blender and mix until smooth.

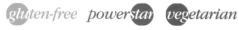 *gluten-free* **powerstar** *vegetarian*

**Per Serving:** Kcal 182, Protein 10g, Carb 34g, Fat 3g, Sodium 120mg, Dietary Fiber 3g
**Daily Values:** Fiber 10%, Vit C 2%, Vit A 10%, Vit D 32%, Calcium 32%, Iron 7%

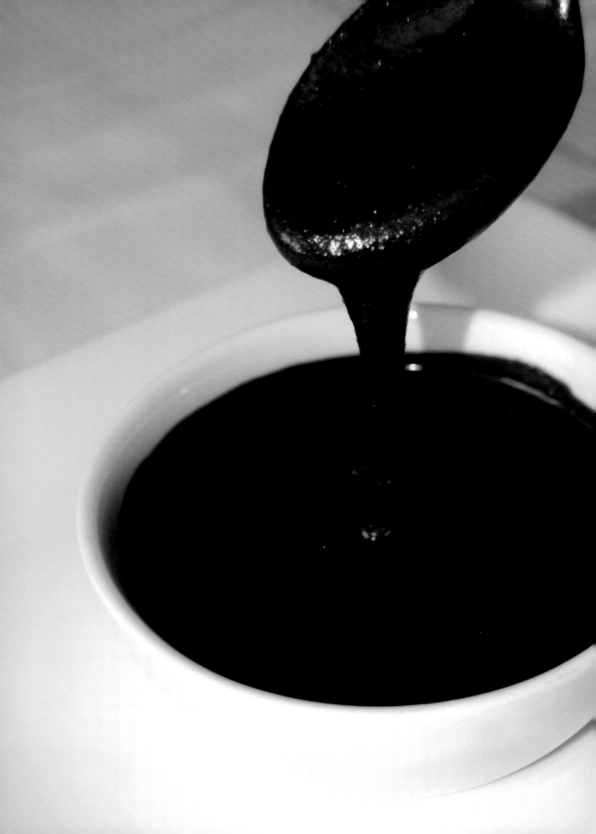

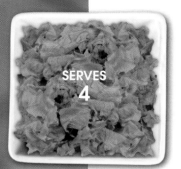

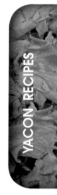

SERVES
4

# YACON CHOCOLATE SYRUP

*This chocolate sauce looks sinful, but with a combination of cacao and yacon, you can feel great about the low glycemic index and high antioxidant power of such a decadent treat.*

## Ingredients

6 tablespoons yacon syrup

1 tablespoon coconut oil

½ cup cacao powder

¼ teaspoon salt

½ teaspoon cinnamon

2 tablespoons water

## Directions

1. In a medium bowl, combine all of the ingredients and mix well with a wire whisk until a smooth sauce forms. Store in an airtight container in the refrigerator for up to a week.

2. Warm the sauce to serve over ice cream, cake, or your favorite dessert.

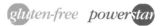 *gluten-free* **power**star *vegan*

**Per Serving:** Kcal 108, Protein 2g, Carb 24g, Fat 5g, Sodium 164mg, Dietary Fiber 3g
**Daily Values:** Fiber 13%, Vit C 0%, Vit A 0%, Vit D 0%, Calcium 2%, Iron 8%

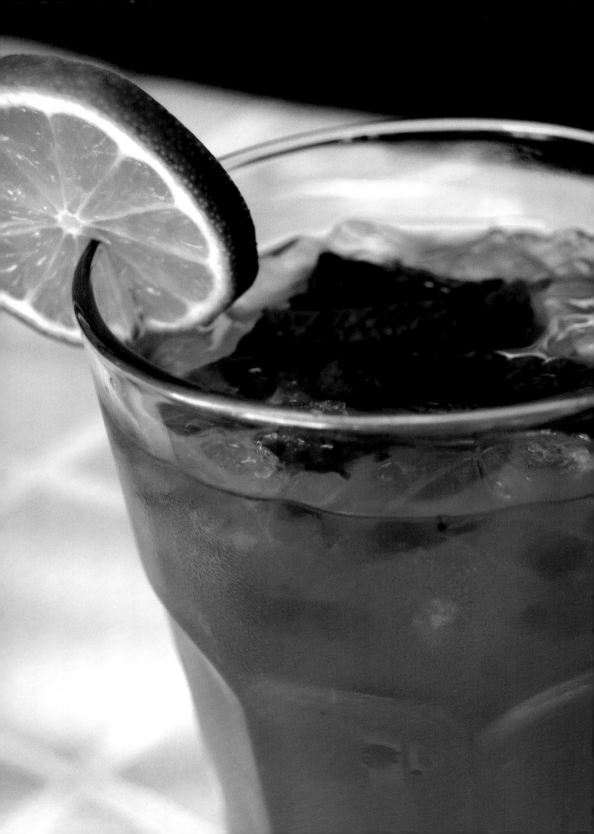

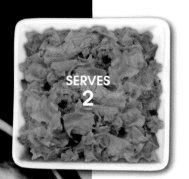

# YACITO COCKTAIL

*Think of this drink as a jungle mojito. This baby is crisp and refreshing with an effervescent fizz.*

**SERVES 2**

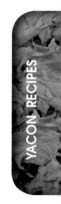
## Ingredients

Handful of ice
8 fresh mint sprigs
3 tablespoons fresh lime juice
3 ounces light rum
2 tablespoons yacon syrup
1 cup club soda
2 slices lime

## Directions

1. In a cocktail shaker, add the ice, 6 muddled (gently crushed) mint sprigs, lime juice, rum, yacon syrup, and club soda. Shake until all of the ingredients and flavors are combined.

2. Fill two glasses with ice and pour the yacito over the ice. Add a fresh mint sprig to each glass and garnish each with a slice of lime.

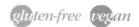

gluten-free  vegan

**Per Serving:** Kcal 252, Protein 0g, Carb 27g, Fat 0g, Sodium 77mg, Dietary Fiber 1g
**Daily Values:** Fiber 2%, Vit C 30%, Vit A 1%, Vit D 0%, Calcium 2%, Iron 3%

# 17 &#x203A; QUINOA

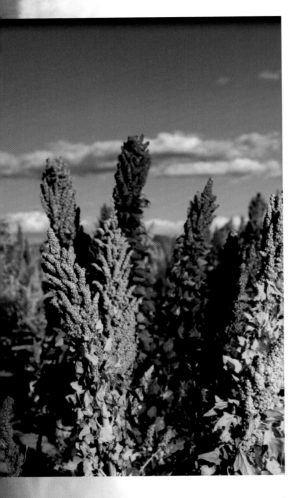

Quinoa has long been a staple of Peruvian cuisine. It is delicious, versatile, and filled with health benefits. The ancient Incas, who discovered the grain, named it "the mother grain" as they believed it was a gift from their gods. The cultivation of quinoa dates back over 5,000 years.

## OVERVIEW

**ALTHOUGH WE COMMONLY** refer to quinoa as a grain, it is technically a seed. And what a seed it is: one-half cup of quinoa contains 340 calories, no saturated fat or cholesterol, 12 grams of protein, 32 grams of carbohydrate, and 10 grams of fiber. In that respect, it's an ideal perfectly balanced food source. Today, quinoa is quite commonplace in our markets and stores, and can even be found in red, white, and black varieties. It's becoming more and more popular for its nutty taste and pleasant, moist texture, not to mention its outstanding nutritional content.

Quinoa is made up of a total of 21 amino acids. Eleven of these can be synthesized by our bodies and are therefore nonessential. However, the 10 remaining essential amino acids make quinoa a complete protein. It's the only seed, or grainlike product, that meets that criterion. Quinoa has a similar protein value to milk, and it's also rich in calcium, copper, iron, magnesium, and zinc.

Quinoa is a fantastic source of fiber—one of the key macronutrients needed for healthy blood-sugar regulation. It also provides outstanding protein quality, even in comparison to commonly eaten whole grains. Strong protein and fiber intake is a dietary essential for regulating blood sugar.

*Quinoa is extremely versatile. We love to make quinoa in advance and then add it to all kinds of different recipes during the week. Toss it in salads, mix it with roasted vegetables, or serve it for breakfast with warm almond milk and blueberries for a protein-packed alternative to oatmeal.*

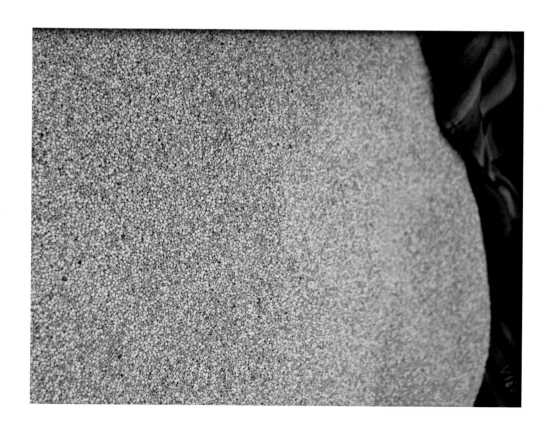

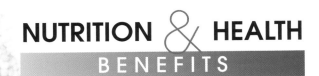

# NUTRITION & HEALTH
## BENEFITS

AIDS WEIGHT LOSS

ANTICANCER

ANTI-INFLAMMATORY

BRAIN HEALTHY

BONE HEALTHY

COMPLETE PROTEIN

HEART HEALTHY

REGULATES BLOOD SUGAR

Quinoa is rich in B vitamins, calcium, copper, iron, magnesium, vitamins C and E, and zinc. Both vitamin E and vitamin C are antioxidants that help prevent free-radical damage. Free radicals are naturally occurring by-products of chemical reactions in the body. However, certain activities, such as consuming a high fat diet and overexposure to sunlight, will increase the amount of free radicals in the body. Left alone, free radicals can cause oxidative damage, which has been linked to many serious conditions, including cancer and heart disease.

Quinoa contains essential fatty acids (EFAs), specifically linoleic acid and linolenic acid. Consuming these polyunsaturated fatty acids has been linked to improved blood sugar control and cardiovascular health.

Quinoa has a very low glycemic index of 35. For people suffering from diabetes, quinoa makes a great carbohydrate source because of the slow rate that it affects blood sugar once eaten.

Regularly consuming certain amino acids, antioxidants, B vitamins, and omega-3s found in quinoa has been associated with increased brain function.

Quinoa is gluten free and lactose free, which makes it a great source of protein for those with Celiac disease or those who are lactose-intolerant or gluten-intolerant.

Quinoa also contains phytosterols, a natural component of their plant cell membranes. Phytosterols have been linked to preventing oxidative damage, preventing cancer growth, and lowering cholesterol. Phytosterols also have anti-inflammatory effects, making quinoa a potentially great food for people experiencing diseases such as arthritis, metabolic syndrome, or the many gastrointestinal inflammatory diseases.

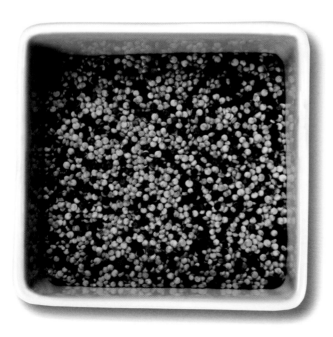

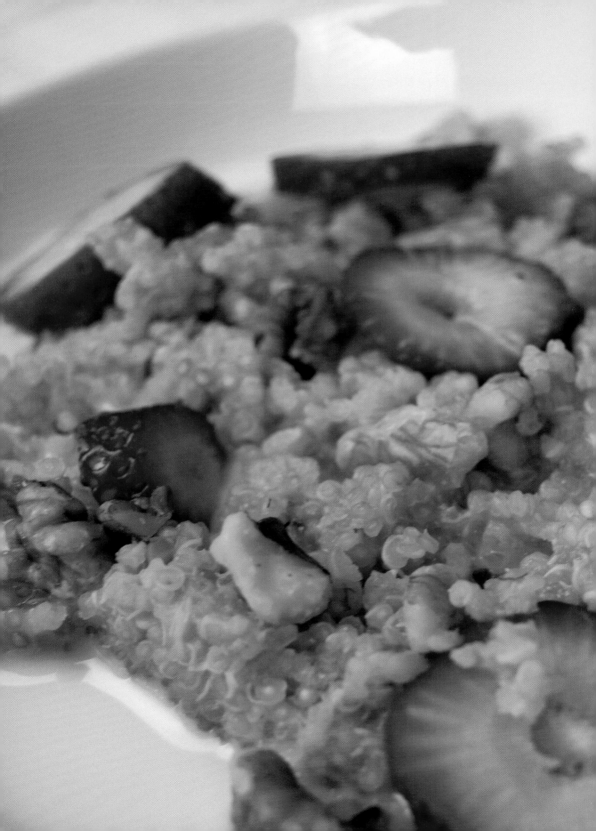

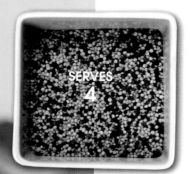

# QUINOA BREX

*We love using quinoa as an alternative to oatmeal. Served warm with fruit or nuts, it's filling, comforting, and delicious—with extra protein to kick-start the day.*

**SERVES 4**

QUINOA RECIPES

## Ingredients

1 cup dry/raw quinoa
2 cups water
1 banana, mashed
1 cinnamon stick
5 cloves
Pinch of salt

## Directions

1. Combine all of the ingredients in a saucepan and stir well. Bring the water to a boil, then cover and reduce the heat to low. Simmer until the quinoa is cooked, roughly 15 minutes. Remove the cinnamon stick and enjoy!

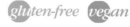 *gluten-free* *vegan*

**Per Serving:** Kcal 197, Protein 7g, Carb 36g, Fat 3g, Sodium 20mg, Dietary Fiber 4g
**Daily Values:** Fiber 17%, Vit C 4%, Vit A 1%, Vit D 0%, Calcium 6%, Iron 13%

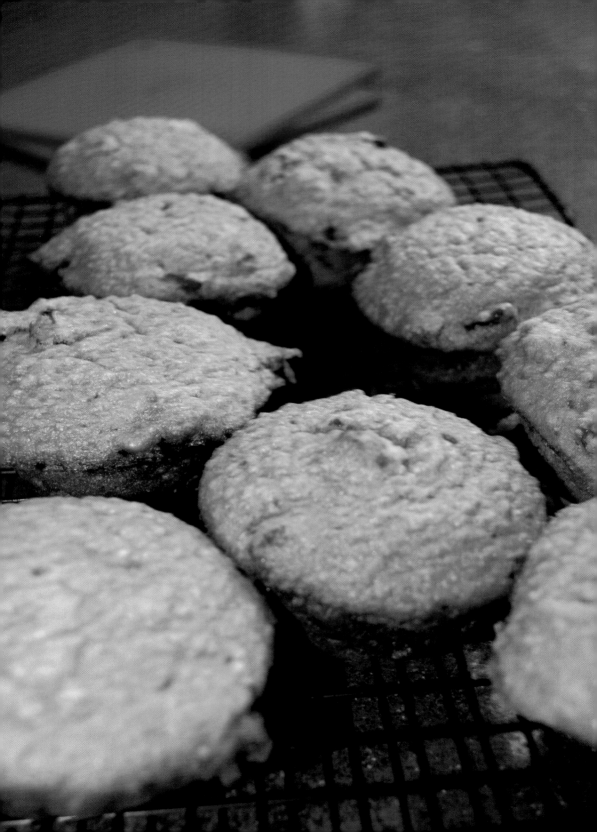

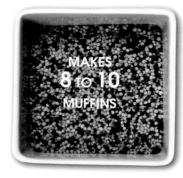

# QUINOA PICHUBERRY MUFFINS

*These muffins are perfect for breakfast or as a grab-and-go snack. We love the dried pichuberries, which add a flavor reminiscent of tart cherry, while the quinoa brings nutty notes and moistens the mix. Plus, quinoa packs these snacks with healthy protein.*

## Ingredients

1⅓ cups applesauce
½ cup agave nectar
2 eggs
½ teaspoon salt
½ teaspoon baking soda

1 teaspoon baking powder
1 cup whole wheat flour
1 cup cooked quinoa
½ cup walnut pieces
1½ cups dried pichuberries

## Directions

1. Preheat the oven to 350 degrees F. In a large bowl, mix the applesauce, agave nectar, eggs, salt, baking soda, and baking powder. Once thoroughly combined, add the whole wheat flour and quinoa. Gently fold in the walnut pieces and dried pichuberries.

2. Lightly spray muffin tins with nonstick spray. Evenly distribute the muffin batter into the tins until they are ½ to ¾ full, depending on your preference. Bake for 30 to 35 minutes, or until the muffins are golden brown and a toothpick inserted in the center comes out clean.

3. Cool in the muffin tray for 5 minutes, and then transfer the muffins to a cooling rack.

**Per Serving:** Kcal 257, Protein 7g, Carb 45g, Fat 6g, Sodium 236mg, Dietary Fiber 5g
**Daily Values:** Fiber 21%, Vit C 4%, Vit A 33%, Vit D 1%, Calcium 5%, Iron 11%

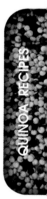
QUINOA RECIPES

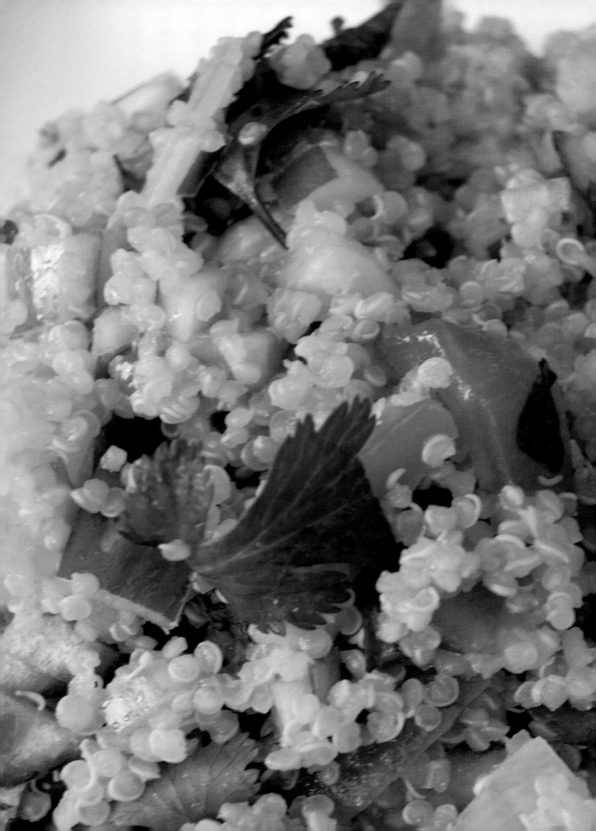

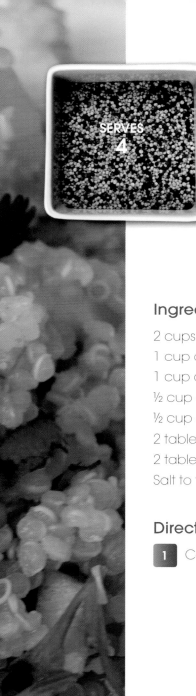

SERVES
4

# PICO DE QUINOA

*Quinoa is a perfect base for all kinds of cold salads, and one of the easiest, most satisfying combinations is this dish, which looks to Mexico for flavor inspiration. If you want an even heartier version, you can crumble some queso fresco on top, or pair with shredded poached chicken.*

## Ingredients

2 cups cooked quinoa
1 cup diced tomato
1 cup diced cucumber
½ cup diced red onion
½ cup chopped cilantro
2 tablespoons lime juice
2 tablespoons sacha inchi oil
Salt to taste

## Directions

1 Combine all of the ingredients in a bowl and enjoy!

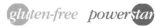 
*gluten-free* **powerstar** *vegan*

Per Serving: Kcal 198, Protein 5g, Carb 25g, Fat 9g, Sodium 11mg, Dietary Fiber 4g
Daily Values: Fiber 15%, Vit C 18%, Vit A 11%, Vit D 0%, Calcium 3%, Iron 9%

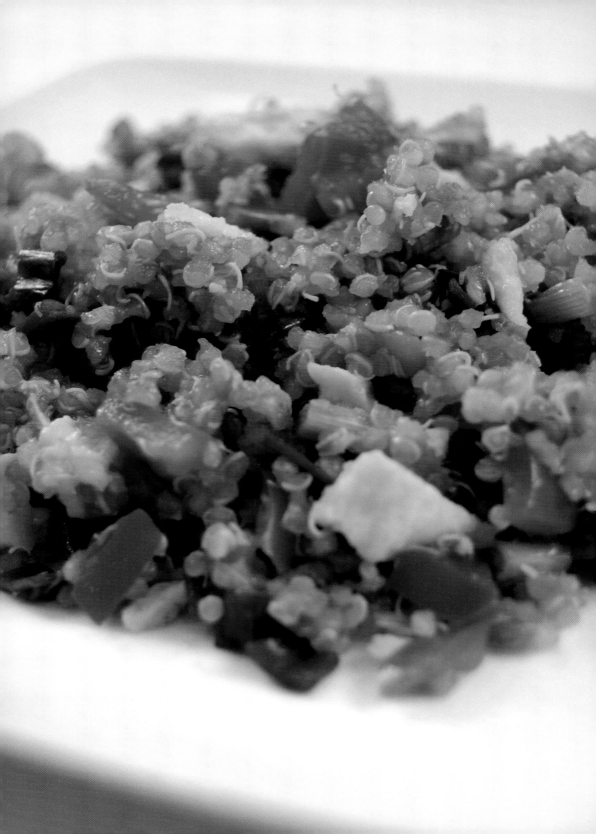

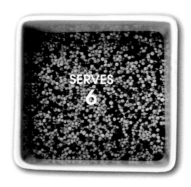

SERVES
6

# QUINOA FRIED RICE

*There's a heavy Asian influence in Peru, notable in the many small restaurants categorized as Chifa, which is a hybrid style of Peruvian and Chinese cuisine. One of the most popular dishes is chaufa, or fried rice, which we've adapted here to be made with protein-rich quinoa.*

## Ingredients

3 eggs

2 tablespoons olive oil

3 cups cooked quinoa

1 bunch scallions, diced and divided
(into the green and white parts)

1 red bell pepper, diced

1 tablespoon ginger, crushed

1 tablespoon garlic, crushed

2 tablespoons soy sauce

## Directions

1. Whisk the eggs together and cook over medium-high heat to make an egg pancake. Once cooked, remove it from the heat, chop into small pieces, and set aside.

2. Heat 2 tablespoons of olive oil in a wok or large frying pan. Add the white parts of the scallion, the red pepper, the ginger, and the garlic. Sauté for roughly 30 seconds to 1 minute. Add the cooked quinoa and sauté for a couple of minutes more, until heated through. Add the green parts of the scallion and the soy sauce, stirring until well heated.

3. Stir in the chopped cooked eggs, and serve.

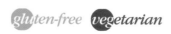

gluten-free  vegetarian

**Per Serving:** Kcal 201, Protein 8g, Carb 23g, Fat 9g, Sodium 382mg, Dietary Fiber 3g
**Daily Values:** Fiber 13%, Vit C 37%, Vit A 14%, Vit D 2%, Calcium 4%, Iron 12%

QUINOA RECIPES

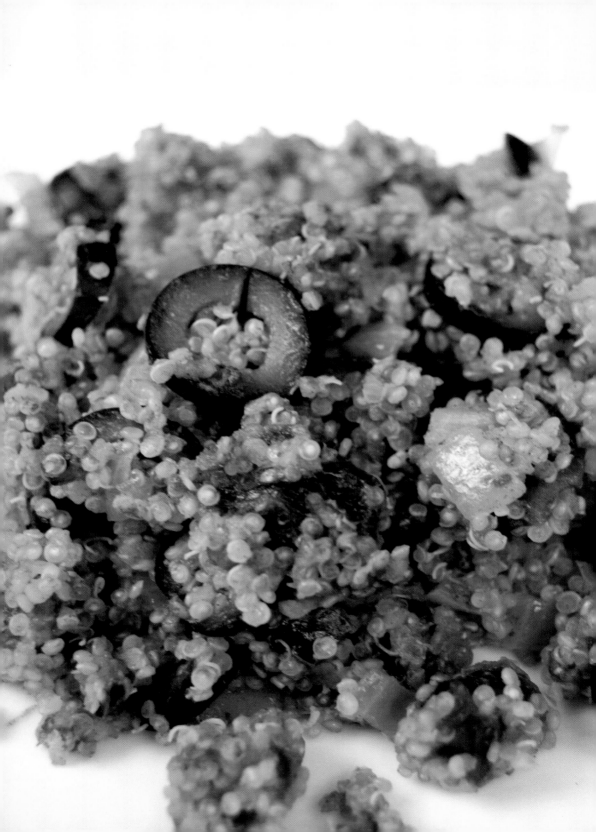

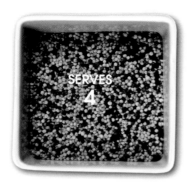

# MIDDLE EASTERN QUINOA

*Because quinoa is so versatile, it serves as the perfect stage to showcase various flavor profiles. Here, we've taken a Moroccan slant with olives and dates, like you might find in a traditional tagine dish.*

**SERVES 4**

## Ingredients

1 small onion, chopped

1 tablespoon olive oil

2 teaspoons minced garlic

1 cup dry/raw quinoa

2 cups vegetable or chicken broth

½ cup sliced black olives

½ cup diced medjool dates

1 tablespoon ground cinnamon

Salt and pepper to taste

## Directions

1. Sauté the onion in olive oil over medium-high heat until the onion is slightly translucent. Add the garlic and sauté an additional minute, or until the garlic is just toasted.

2. Add the quinoa to the onions and brown while stirring, roughly 3 minutes.

3. Add the broth and bring to a boil. Reduce the heat to simmer and cover and cook for roughly 15 minutes, or until the quinoa is fully cooked.

4. Remove from the heat and gently fold in the olives and dates. Garnish with the cinnamon and season with the salt and pepper to taste.

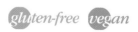 *gluten-free* *vegan*

**Per Serving:** Kcal 294, Protein 7g, Carb 51g, Fat 8g, Sodium 380mg, Dietary Fiber 7g
**Daily Values:** Fiber 27%, Vit C 4%, Vit A 12%, Vit D 0%, Calcium 8%, Iron 17%

QUINOA RECIPES

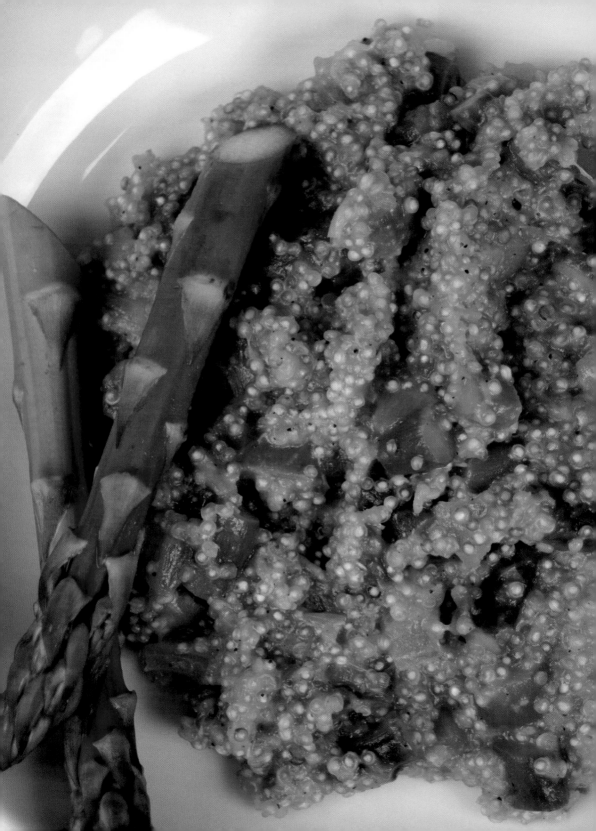

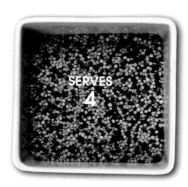

SERVES
4

# QUINOA RISOTTO WITH ASPARAGUS

*Learning that we could use quinoa as a substitute for Arborio rice in risotto was an inspired discovery. You can enjoy all the creamy, cheesy goodness of a heart-comforting dish with added nutritional value and a whole protein base. Buon appetito!*

## Ingredients

1½ cups asparagus, thinly sliced
  on the diagonal
2 tablespoons olive oil
1 teaspoon each salt and pepper
1 medium onion, diced

3 cloves garlic, minced
1 cup dry/raw quinoa
2 cups vegetable or chicken stock
2 ounces shredded Parmesan
  cheese

## Directions

1  In a medium saucepan, sauté the asparagus in olive oil over medium-high heat, roughly 2 to 3 minutes. Season with the salt and pepper. Add the onion to the pan and cook until translucent. Add the garlic and sauté an additional minute. Be careful not to let the garlic brown and burn. Add the quinoa and lightly toast until golden brown, about 2 to 3 minutes. Add the stock and allow the mixture to come to a boil. Cover and reduce the heat to low.

2  Simmer until the quinoa is cooked, about 15 minutes. Do not overcook the quinoa; you want it to have a bite and be al dente.

3  Add the Parmesan cheese just before removing the quinoa from the heat.

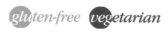 gluten-free vegetarian

**Per Serving:** Kcal 316, Protein 13g, Carb 36g, Fat 14g, Sodium 451mg, Dietary Fiber 5g
**Daily Values:** Fiber 20%, Vit C 9%, Vit A 19%, Vit D 1%, Calcium 21%, Iron 19%

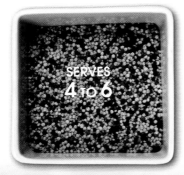

SERVES
4 to 6

# QUINOA CAULIFLOWER PIZZA CRUST

*We love pizza, and we knew we wanted to include a gluten-free, quinoa-based option. We'd also been experimenting with using cauliflower in the crust. It took three tries, but we finally landed on a winner. This crust is fantastic, and it leaves you wanting for nothing, despite its healthy content.*

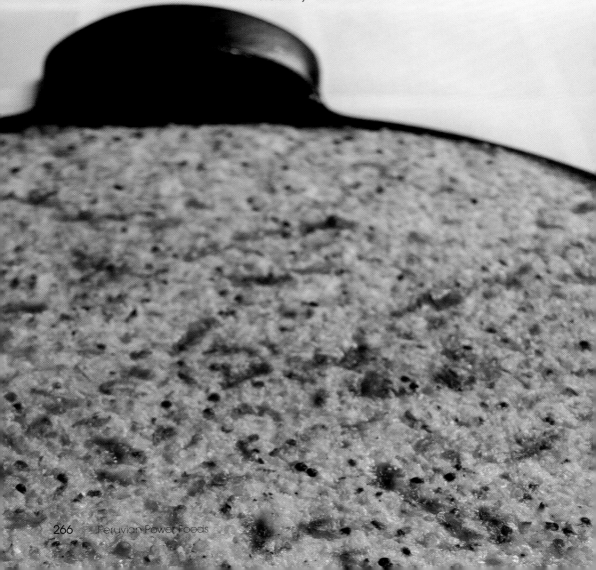

## Ingredients

2 cups raw cauliflower

1 cup cooked quinoa

½ cup shredded Parmesan cheese

½ cup 2% plain Greek yogurt

½ cup egg whites

1 tablespoon dried oregano

1 teaspoon each salt and pepper

4 tablespoons tomato sauce

8 ounces shredded mozzarella cheese

Toppings of choice

## Directions

**1** Preheat the oven to 400 degrees F, and place the oven rack in the middle.

**2** In a food processor, pulse the cauliflower until it looks like small grains of orzo.

**3** In a large bowl, combine the cauliflower, quinoa, Parmesan cheese, Greek yogurt, egg whites, oregano, and salt and pepper. Mix until thoroughly combined. Transfer the mixture to a lightly greased pizza stone and spread evenly with a spatula or your hands.

**4** Bake for 20 minutes, or until the crust is crispy and golden brown. Remove from the oven and allow to slightly cool.

**5** Increase the oven temperature to broil (500 degrees F) and move the oven rack up one level, about 7 to 8 inches away from broiler.

**6** Spread the tomato sauce evenly over the pizza crust with a brush or a spatula. Add the mozzarella cheese and toppings of choice (we used chicken sausage, tomato, and red onion). Bake until the cheese is melted and the toppings are thoroughly heated.

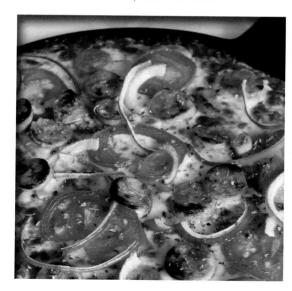

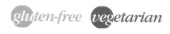

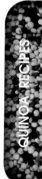

Per Serving: Kcal 247, Protein 23g, Carb 13g, Fat 11g, Sodium 271mg, Dietary Fiber 2g
Daily Values: Fiber 9%, Vit C 32%, Vit A 8%, Vit D 0%, Calcium 48%, Iron 6%

# 18 ⌒ SWEET POTATOES

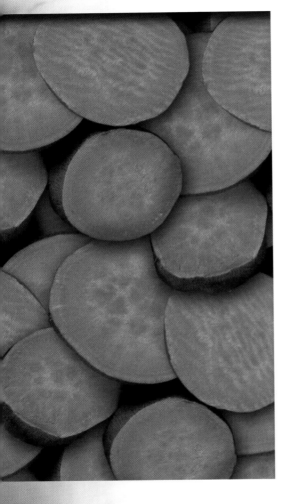

## OVERVIEW

**SWEET POTATOES ARE EASILY** distinguished from yellow potatoes by their pale purple skins, bright orange flesh, and elongated rootlike shape. The biggest clue to their health benefits comes through their color. In the case of sweet potatoes, the color is attributable to a high level of beta-carotene. Besides supporting eye health, sweet potatoes scavenge free radicals, which can cause cancer.

The domestication of sweet potatoes in Peru can be traced back 5,000 years. In fact, ancient ceramics found in Peruvian tombs depict renderings of sweet potatoes, signaling their importance in early civilization.

While the sweet potato is a common staple in Peru, we notice that in America, it gets a brief nod around Thanksgiving, and then it's often whipped into sugary creations with marshmallows and bourbon. We hope this power-packed tuber will gain acceptance and find a place in more Americans' regular diets—it's so delicious and full of health benefits.

*Sweet potatoes are delicious eaten simply baked, but in Peruvian cuisine they are used in a vast array of dishes in preparations ranging from stews and baked fries, to mousses, steamed accompaniments, and ceviches.*

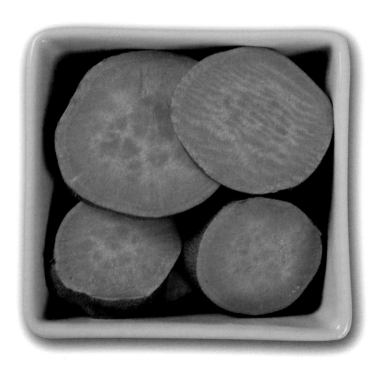

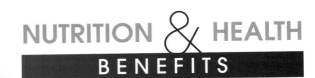

# NUTRITION & HEALTH
## BENEFITS

ANTICANCER

HEART HEALTHY

IMMUNE SYSTEM BOOSTER

SUPPORTS EYE HEALTH

Nutritionally, sweet potatoes are very high in beta-carotene, calcium, iron, and vitamins A and C. The vitamin A content far exceeds daily requirements.

Touted as the next miracle anti-aging solution, sweet potatoes have properties that fight wrinkle formation and promote soft, youthful skin.

Sweet potatoes are also potent free-radical scavengers that prevent DNA damage at the cellular level, helping to prevent disease and to slow aging.

Sweet potatoes are rich in beta-carotene, a powerful antioxidant that has been shown to prevent oxidative damage, which can help prevent both cancer and cardiovascular disease. It also shows potential to specifically fight oral, pharynx, and larynx cancers.

Consuming large amounts of beta-carotene reduces the risk of cataracts and macular degeneration.

Research shows that beta-carotene can lower the risk of heart attack in men.

Sweet potatoes are packed with vitamin C, which helps prevent lung cancer in smokers and helps decrease the mortality rate of those with lung cancer.

Vitamin C supports immune system health, inhibits tumor spread and metastases, and decreases the risk of coronary heart disease.

Vitamin C has been strongly linked to a decreased risk of many types of cancer, including oral, esophageal, stomach, pancreatic, cervical, and rectal.

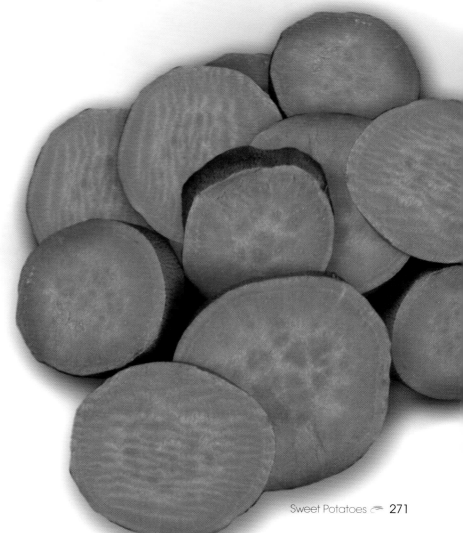

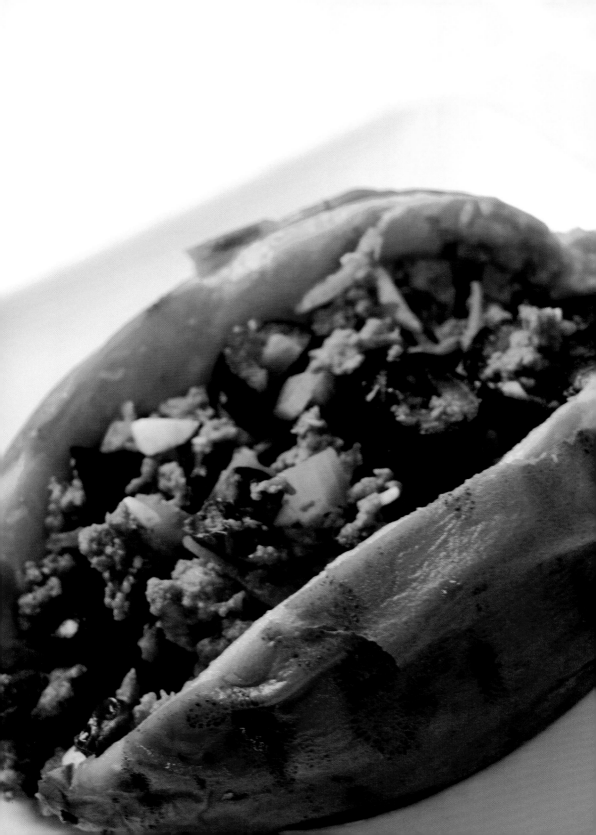

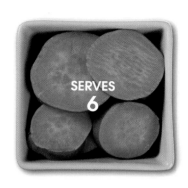

**SERVES 6**

# SWEET POTATO WITH EMPANADA BEEF STUFFING

*One of the most popular foods across South America is the empanada. We love the combination of piquant olives and sweet currants with beef and egg. In our version, we replaced the flaky dough casing with a sweet potato bowl. It's a healthier take on the classic, and it adds another dimension of flavor and texture that beautifully complements the filling.*

## Ingredients

6 sweet potatoes, baked

1 tablespoon olive oil

1 onion, chopped

3 cloves garlic, minced

1 pound lean ground beef

1 cup black olives, sliced (you can also use green if you prefer)

2 hard-boiled eggs, chopped

½ cup currants or raisins

## Directions

1. Preheat the oven to 400 F. Wrap the sweet potatoes in foil and prick the wrapped potatoes with a fork. Bake for 45 minutes, remove from the oven, and carefully unwrap. Set them aside while you prepare the empanada stuffing.

2. Sauté the onions and garlic until the onions are soft and translucent. Add the ground beef to the pan and brown it. Add the olives, eggs, and currants or raisins to the pan, mix well, and thoroughly cook, approximately 20 minutes.

3. Cut the sweet potatoes in half, mash up the flesh, and scoop a bit of flesh out to create a "bowl" in the middle. Add the empanada stuffing to each sweet potato half. Serve immediately.

**SWEET POTATO RECIPES**

**Per Serving:** Kcal 383, Protein 23g, Carb 51g, Fat 11g, Sodium 333mg, Dietary Fiber 7g
**Daily Values:** Fiber 30%, Vit C 63%, Vit A 4%, Vit D 2%, Calcium 12%, Iron 24%

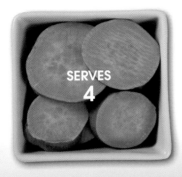

# SWEET POTATO GNOCCHI

*Light and airy with a delicate flavor, this is a great dish for lunch or dinner. Gnocchi can be made in advance and refrigerated until serving time. You can serve them with almost any herb butter, but we think sage butter is especially wonderful. This recipe comes to us from chef Morena Cuadra from PeruDelights.*

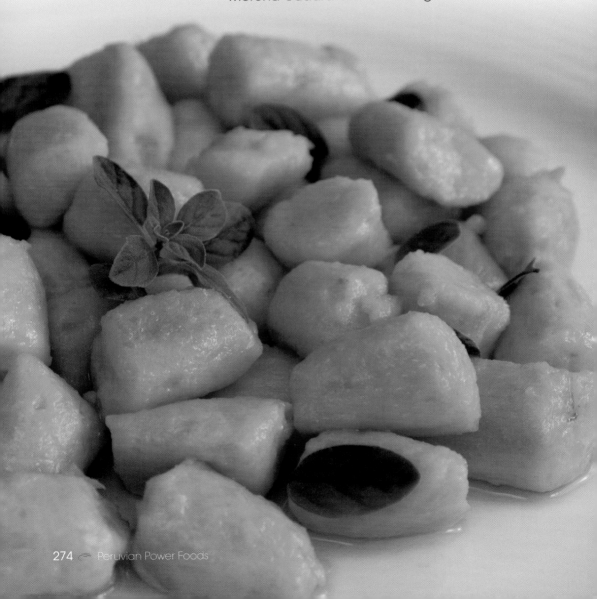

## Ingredients

½ cup milk

¼ cup butter

½ teaspoon salt

½ cup all-purpose flour

3 eggs

2 cups sweet potato, boiled until tender and pureed

⅓ cup crumbled goat cheese or grated Parmesan cheese

Salt and pepper to taste

½ cup butter

4 tablespoons fresh herbs (fresh oregano, tarragon, chives, or sage)

## Directions

**1** Heat the milk, butter, and salt in a small saucepan over medium heat. Bring to a boil and add the flour, stirring constantly until the mixture is smooth and doesn't stick to the sides of the pan. Turn off the heat. Add one egg at a time, stirring with a wooden spoon until incorporated. Add the sweet potato puree and goat cheese, and season with salt and pepper.

**2** Spoon the potato mixture gently into a pastry bag. Set aside (upright in a mug works well) and start a pot of water boiling.

**3** Using a pastry bag with a round tip, form the gnocchi lengths about ¾ of an inch long; drop the gnocchi in gently boiling salted water, and cook until they float, approximately 5 minutes. Drain. Keep them refrigerated in a sealed container.

**4** To serve: in a skillet, heat the remaining butter until very hot, add the gnocchi, and stir-fry until lightly brown and fragrant.

**5** Garnish with fresh herbs and serve immediately.

*vegetarian*

**Per Serving:** Kcal 466, Protein 14g, Carb 43g, Fat 27g, Sodium 495mg, Dietary Fiber 5g
**Daily Values:** Fiber 18%, Vit C 38%, Vit A 540%, Vit D 10%, Calcium 16%, Iron 16%

SWEET POTATO RECIPES

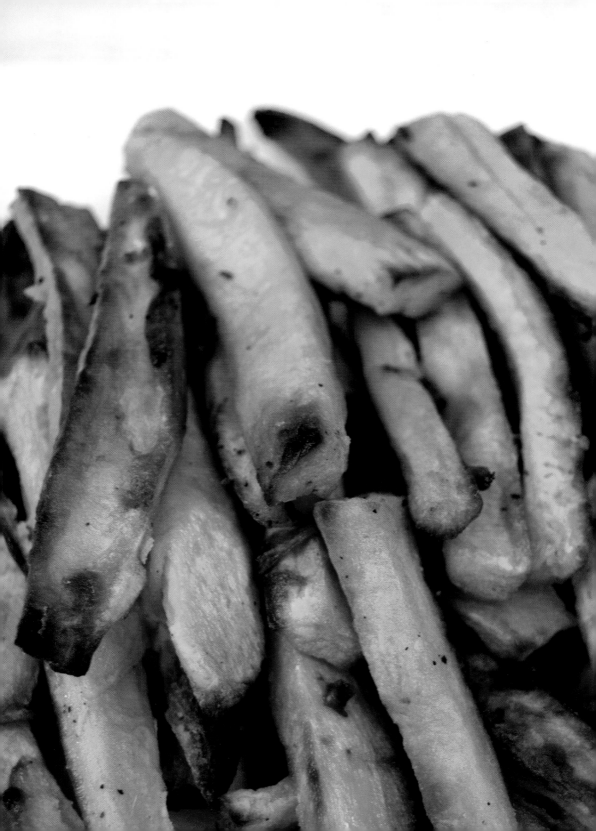

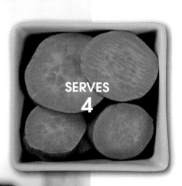

# BAKED SWEET POTATO STICKS

*If you love fries, but you want a healthier alternative, try this baked version that uses sweet potatoes. You'll get all the power-food benefits with none of the fat from frying.*

## Ingredients

1 pound sweet potatoes, cleaned and peeled
2 tablespoons olive oil
Salt to taste

## Directions

1. Preheat the oven to 400 degrees F.

2. Cut the potatoes into 3- to 4-inch strips lengthwise to create "sticks." Toss the potatoes in a bowl with the olive oil to coat.

3. Layer the sticks on a baking sheet or roasting pan and season with salt. Bake for 20 to 25 minutes, or until the fries are crispy and golden brown.

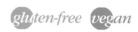 gluten-free vegan

**Per Serving:** Kcal 157, Protein 2g, Carb 23g, Fat 7g, Sodium 63mg, Dietary Fiber 3g
**Daily Values:** Fiber 14%, Vit C 5%, Vit A 322%, Vit D 0%, Calcium 3%, Iron 4%

Sweet Potatoes 277

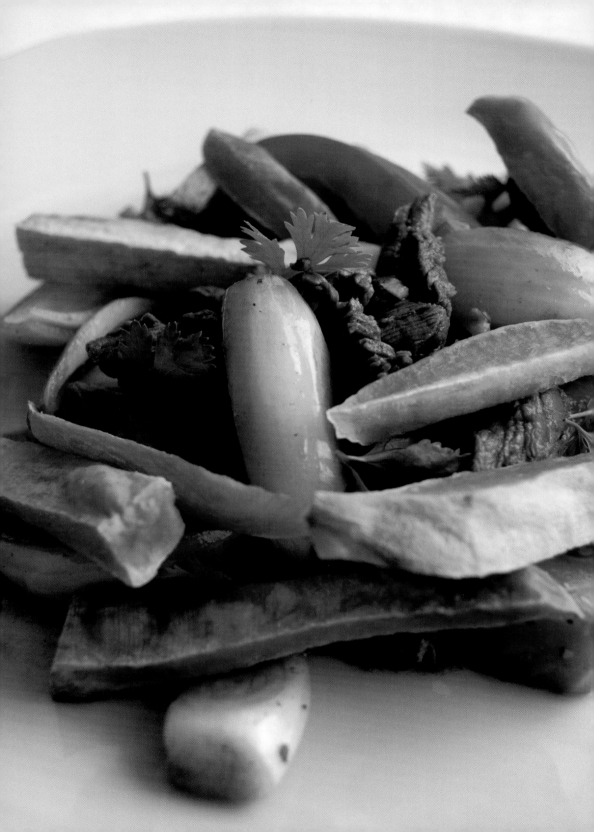

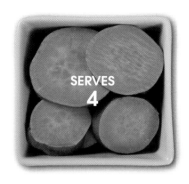

# LOMO SALTADO WITH SWEET POTATO STICKS

**SERVES 4**

Lomo saltado, *which is a beef stir-fry, is a very popular dish in Peru. It is obviously Asian influenced and is commonly found in the ubiquitous Chifa (Peruvian-Chinese) restaurants as well as in many home kitchens. Here, we present a standard home recipe for* lomo saltado *with the addition of healthy sweet potato sticks as an accompaniment.*

## Ingredients

2 tablespoons olive oil

1 pound beef tri-tip or filet mignon,
   thinly sliced into stick-shaped pieces

Salt and pepper to taste

1 to 2 teaspoons of cumin to taste

2 red onions, cut into "sticks"

1 clove garlic, minced

1 tablespoon aji sauce

2 tablespoons balsamic vinegar

2 tomatoes, cut into "sticks"

3 tablespoons soy sauce

2 tablespoons chopped cilantro

1 pound baked sweet potato sticks
   (see page 277)

## Directions

1. Heat the oil and sauté the meat in a pan. Season with salt and pepper and stir in the cumin. Remove the meat from the pan.

2. Add the onions, garlic, aji, and vinegar to the pan. Cook for 2 to 3 minutes. Add the tomatoes and mix well. Return the beef to the pan, add the soy sauce, and sprinkle with cilantro. Stir.

3. Place the sweet potato sticks on top of each serving of the beef mixture and serve immediately.

**SWEET POTATO RECIPES**

**Per Serving:** Kcal 416, Protein 28g, Carb 34g, Fat 18g, Sodium 806mg, Dietary Fiber 6g
**Daily Values:** Fiber 22%, Vit C 57%, Vit A 448%, Vit D 0%, Calcium 11%, Iron 17%

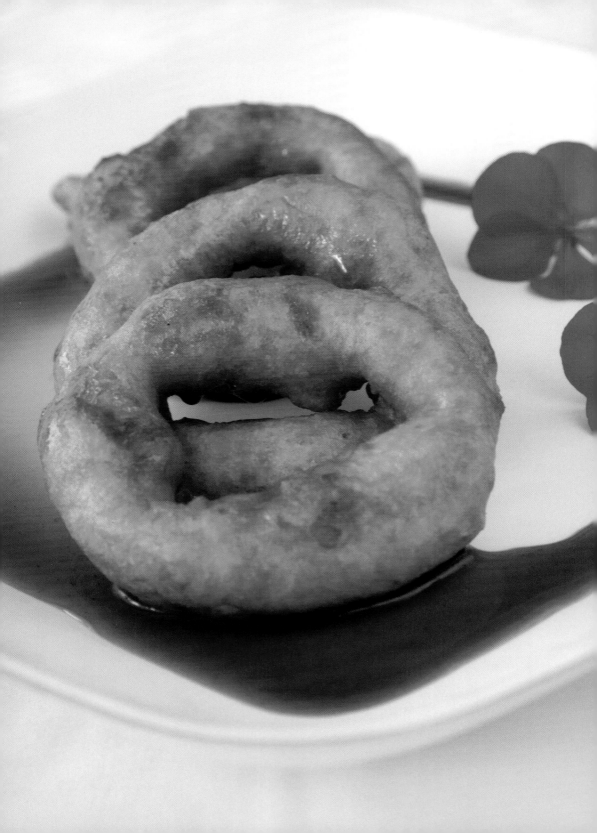

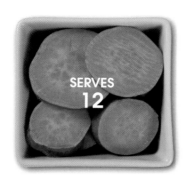

# PICARONES

*Think of these delicious traditional fritters as Peruvian doughnuts—just made with sweet potatoes and pumpkin. We asked chef Morena Cuadra from* PeruDelights *to share a family recipe as she specializes in traditional foods, and this is a Peruvian classic.*

*The dough should be prepared in advance because the yeast needs time to work its magic. A word of advice: picarones must be eaten as soon as they are fried, otherwise they will be soggy and unappetizing. Serve hot with* chancaca, *an anise-infused syrup, or yacon or agave syrups.*

## Ingredients

**For picarones:**

1 pound sweet potatoes, peeled and diced

1 pound pumpkin, peeled and diced

2 teaspoons aniseed

1 tablespoon sugar

½ teaspoon salt

1½ tablespoons active dry yeast (or use instant yeast to make it faster)

4 cups all-purpose flour

Vegetable oil for frying

**For chancaca syrup (makes 3 cups):**

2 chancaca pieces, chopped

2 cinnamon sticks

4 cloves

2 star anise

Peel of 1 pineapple

1 quince, chopped

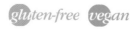

*gluten-free* *vegan*

**SWEET POTATO RECIPES**

**Per Serving:** Kcal 205, Protein 6g, Carb 44g, Fat 11g, Sodium 113mg, Dietary Fiber 3g
**Daily Values:** Fiber 12%, Vit C 18%, Vit A 201%, Vit D 0%, Calcium 3%, Iron 16%

# Directions

**For picarones:**

**1**   Put the sweet potatoes and pumpkin in a heavy saucepan with the aniseed; add enough water to cover, and cook over medium-high heat until soft. Drain the sweet potatoes and pumpkin. Reserve the water and set aside. Transfer the potatoes and pumpkin to the bowl of a food processor, and process to form a soft puree.

**2**   When the cooking water is lukewarm, measure out one cup and place it in a bowl with the sugar and salt (reserve the remaining cooking liquid). Add the active dry yeast, stirring until dissolved. Cover with a kitchen cloth and let the mixture rest for 10 minutes in a warm place, until it forms a sponge-like consistency.

**3**   Transfer the potato and pumpkin puree to a large bowl and add the activated yeast. Add the flour and ½ cup of the reserved cooking water. Mix the dough with your hands until it is no longer sticky and feels soft and silky. Cover the bowl with a kitchen towel and let it rest in a warm place until the dough doubles or triples in volume, about 1 or 2 hours.

**4**   When you are ready to cook the picarones, heat a good amount of oil in a big saucepan to deep-fry the dough. This step requires a little practice, so don't be discouraged if your first rings look more like fritters. Wet your hands with cold water, take a portion of the dough, and try to quickly make a ring shape, using your thumb to poke a hole in the center just as you drop the dough in the hot oil. You can try 2 or 3 at a time, depending on the size. With a long wooden spoon, turn the picarones and cook the other side until nicely brown. Serve with chancaca syrup.

**For chancaca syrup:**

**1**   In a saucepan over medium heat, combine all of the ingredients with water to cover. Simmer, stirring occasionally, until the syrup thickens lightly. It should have the texture of maple syrup. Strain and discard the spices and fruits. Cool to room temperature before serving.

# CONCLUSION

**WE HOPE YOU HAVE ENJOYED** experimenting with new foods and recipes as much as we have. By bringing these Peruvian power foods to your plate you'll enjoy great meals with flavor and flair, as well as improved health and vitality. Salud!

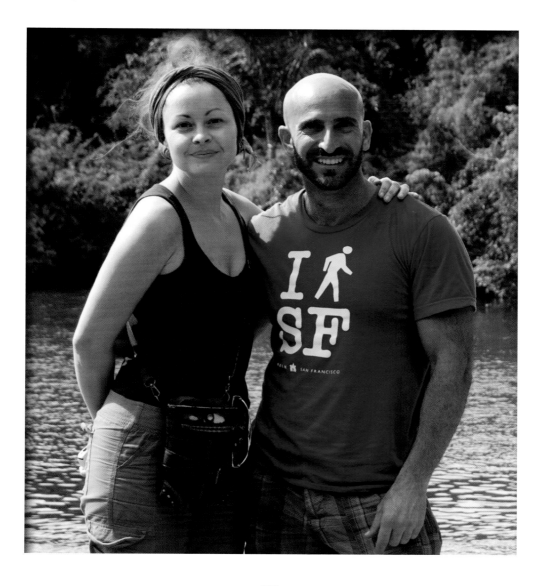

# APPENDIX A

## Recipes by Meal Type

### STARTERS & SIDES

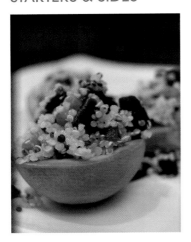

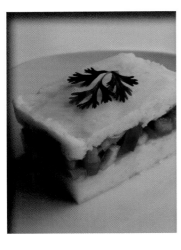

## BREAKFAST

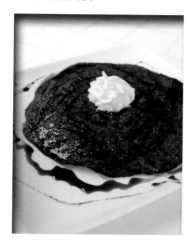

## LUNCH/DINNER

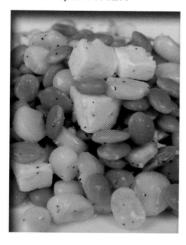

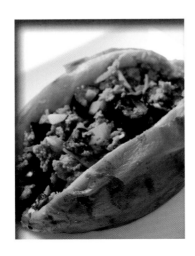

## DESSERTS

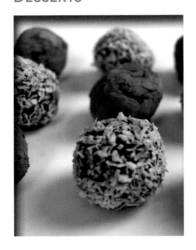

## SMOOTHIES

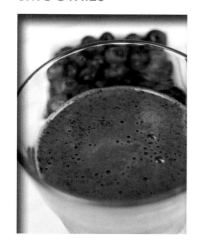

## DRINKS, COFFEE DRINKS & COCKTAILS

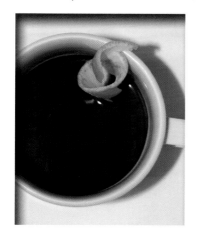

## SNACKS

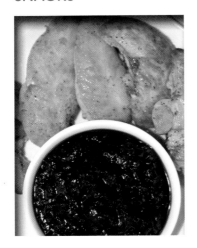

## DRESSINGS & SAUCES

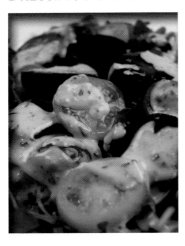

# 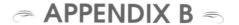 APPENDIX B

## Online Resources

To make things easy, check **EatingFree.com** and **PeruvianPowerFoods.com** before hunting around online. These two sites carry a good many of the power foods we reference, so they're a good starting point. Many of these foods are now carried in health food stores, Latino markets and/or regular supermarkets like Whole Foods, Trader Joe's, Safeway, Publix, and General Markets.

Brands used were Sacha Vida, Navitas, Barry Farm, and Bobs Red Mill.

To learn more, connect with us on the social media sites listed below. We will be routinely updating these sites with more nutrition info, recipes, cooking tips, videos, and future power foods.

Facebook: https://www.facebook.com/EatingFree

Twitter: https://twitter.com/EatingFree

Pinterest: http://pinterest.com/eatingfree/

# METRIC CONVERSION GUIDE

## VOLUME

| US Units | | US Units | |
|---|---|---|---|
| ¼ teaspoon | 1 mL | ¾ cup | 175 mL |
| ½ teaspoon | 2 mL | 1 cup | 250 mL |
| 1 teaspoon | 5 mL | 1 quart | 1 liter |
| 1 tablespoon | 15 mL | 1½ quarts | 1.5 liters |
| ¼ cup | 50 mL | 2 quarts | 2 liters |
| ⅓ cup | 75 mL | 2½ quarts | 2.5 liters |
| ½ cup | 125 mL | 3 quarts | 3 liters |
| ⅔ cup | 150 mL | 4 quarts | 4 liters |

## WEIGHT

| US Units | | US Units | |
|---|---|---|---|
| 1 ounce | 30 grams | 8 ounces | 225 grams |
| 3 ounces | 85 grams | 12 ounces | 360 grams |
| 4 ounces | 115 grams | 16 ounces | 455 grams |

## MEASUREMENTS

| Inches | Centimeters | Inches | Centimeters |
|---|---|---|---|
| 1 | 2.5 | 8 | 20.5 |
| 2 | 5.0 | 9 | 23.0 |
| 3 | 7.5 | 10 | 25.5 |
| 4 | 10.0 | 11 | 28.0 |
| 5 | 12.5 | 12 | 30.5 |
| 6 | 15.0 | 13 | 33.0 |
| 7 | 17.5 | | |

# TEMPERATURE

| Fahrenheit | Celsius |
|---|---|
| 32° | 0° |
| 212° | 100° |
| 250° | 120° |
| 275° | 140° |
| 300° | 150° |
| 325° | 160° |
| 350° | 180° |
| 375° | 190° |
| 400° | 200° |
| 425° | 220° |
| 450° | 230° |

# PAN SIZES

|  | Inches | Metric Volume | Centimeters |
|---|---|---|---|
| Baking Pan | 8 x 8 x 2 | 2 L | 20 x 20 x 5 |
| Cake Pan | 9 x 9 x 2 | 2.5 L | 23 x 23 x 5 |
| Loaf Pan | 8 x 4 x 3 | 1.5 L | 20 x 10 x 7 |
|  | 9 x 5 x 3 | 2 L | 23 x 13 x 7 |
| Round Pan | 8 x 1½ | 1.2 L | 20 x 4 |
|  | 9 x 1¼ | 1.5 L | 23 x 4 |
| Pie Plate | 8 x 1¼ | 750 mL | 20 x 3 |
|  | 9 x 1¼ | 1 L | 23 x 3 |

*The recipes in this cookbook were not developed or tested using metric conversions. When converting recipes to metric, some variations in quality may be noticed.*

# ☙ REFERENCES ☙

## CHAPTER 1: PICHUBERRY

Aggarwal, B., Ichikawa, H., Jayaprakasam, B., Nair, M., Shishodia, T., Takada, Y. (2006). Withanolides potentiate apoptosis, inhibit invasion, and abolish osteoclastogenesis through suppression of nuclear factor-KB (NF-KB) activation and NF-KB-regulated gene expression. *Molecular Cancer Therapeutics.* 5.

Arun, M. & Asha, V. V. (2007). Preliminary studies on antihepatotoxic effect of *Physalis peruviana* Linn. (Solanaceae) against carbon tetrachloride induced acute liver injury in rats. *Journal of Ethnopharmacology,* 111, 110–14.

Fang, S. T., Liu, J. K., & Li, B. (2012). Ten new withanolides from *Physalis peruviana. Steroids,* 77, 36–44.

Fischer, G., Ebert., G. & Ludders, P. (2000). Provitamin A carotenoids, organic acids and ascorbic acid content of cape gooseberry (*Physalis peruviana* L.) ecotypes grown at two tropical altitudes. *Acta Hort.,* 351, 263–68.

Franco, L. A., Matiz, G. E., Calle, J., Pinzon, R., & Ospina, L. F. (2007). Actividad antinflamatoria de extractos y fracciones obtenidas de calices de *Physalis peruviana* L. *Biomedica,* 47 (1), 51–60.

Martinez, W. Ospina, L. F., Granados, D., & Delago, G. (2010). In vitro studies on the relationship between the anti-inflammatory activity of *Physalis peruviana* extracts and the phagocytic process. *Immunopharmacology and Immunotoxicology,* 32 (1), 63–73.

Puente, L. A, Pinto-Munoz, C. A., Castro, E. S., & Cortes, M. (2011). *Physalis peruviana* Linnaeus, the multiple properties of a highly functional fruit: A review. *Food Research International,* 44, 1733–40.

Ramadan, M. F. & Morsel, J. T. (2005). Cape gooseberry: a golden fruit of golden future. *Fruit Processing,* 15 (6), 396–400.

Ramadan, M. F. & Morsel, J. T. (2003). Oil Goldenberry (*Physalis peruviana* L.). *Journal of Agriculture and Food Chemistry,* 51 (4), 969–74.

Rockenbach, I. I., et al. (2008). Phenolic acids and antioxidant activity of *Physalis peruviana* L. fruit. *Alimentos e Nutricao,* 19 (3), 271–76.

Wu, S. J., et al. (2005). Antioxidant activities of *Physalis peruviana. Biological Pharmaceutical Bulletin,* 28 (6), 963–66.

Yen, C. Y., et al. (2010). 4B-Hydroxywithanolide E from *Physalis peruviana* (golden berry) inhibits growth of human lung cancer cells through DNA damage, apoptosis and G2/M arrest. *BMC Cancer,* 10 (46).

## CHAPTER 2: MACA

Angeles, F., Condezo, L., Lao, J., Melchor, V., Miller, M., Okuhama, N., Sandoval, M.

(2001). Antioxidant activity of cruciferous vegetable Maca (*Lepidium meyenii*). *Food Chemistry.* 79 (2).

Bianchi, A. (2003). MACA *Lepidium meyenii. Boletín Latinoamericano y del Caribe de Plantas Medicinales y Aromáticas,* 2 (3).

Cordova, A., Chung, A., Gonzales, C., Gonzales, G., Vega, K., & Villena, A. *Lepidium meyenii* (maca) improved semen parameters in adult men. (2001). *Asian Journal of Andrology.* 3.

Gonzales-Castaneda, C., Gonzales, C., & Gonzales, G. F. *Lepidium meyenii* (Maca): A plant from the highlands of Peru—from tradition to science (Abstract). (2009) *Research in Complementary Medicine,* 16 (6).

Gonzales, G. (2011). Ethnobiology and Ethnopharmacology of *Lepidium meyenii* (Maca), a Plant from the Peruvian Highlands. *Evidence-Based Complementary and Alternative Medicine,* Volume 2012.

Kilham, C. (n,d). Maca: peru's natural viagra. Retrieved from: http://health.discovery.com/sex/libido/maca.html.

Sandoval, M., et al., (2002). Antioxidant activity of the cruciferous vegetable Maca (*Lepdidium meyenii*). *Food Chemistry,* 79, 207–13.

Taylor, L. (2005). Maca *(Lepidium meyenii)*. Retrieved from: http://www.rain-tree.com/maca.html.

Wang, Y., et al, Maca: An Andean crop with multi-pharmacological functions. *Food Research International,* 40, 783–92.

## CHAPTER 3: CACAO

Andújar, M., Giner, R. M., Recio, M. C., & Ríos, J. L. Cocoa polyphenols and their potential benefits for human health. (2012). *Oxidative Medicine and Cellular Longevity,* Volume 2012.

Ismail, A. & Jalil, A. M. M. (2008). Polyphenols in cocoa and cocoa products: Is there a link between antioxidant properties and health? *Molecules,* 13 (9), 2190–219.

## CHAPTER 4: KIWICHA

Amaya-Farfán, J. & Caselato-Sousa, V. State of knowledge on amaranth grain: A comprehensive review. (2012). *Journal of Food Science,* 77 (4).

Bavec, F., Bavec, M., Jakop, M., Mlakar, S., & Turinek, M. (2010). Grain amaranth as an alternative perspective crop in temperate climate. *Journal of Geography,* 5 (1), 135–45.

## CHAPTER 5: AVOCADO

Byrns, R., Gao, K., Heber, D., Lee, R., Lu, Q., Wang, D., Wang, Y., & Zhang, Y. (2010). California Hass Avocado: Profiling of carotenoids, tocopherol, fatty acid, and fat content during maturation and from different growing areas. *Journal of Agricultural and Food Chemistry,* 57, 10408–13.

Chin, Y. W., D'Ambrosio, S. M., Ding, H., & Kinghorn, A. D. (2007). Chemopreventative characteristics of avocado fruit. *Seminars in Cancer Biology*, 17, 386–94.

Domínguez, H., Juárez, C., Ledesma, L., Luna, H., Montalvo, C., Morán, L., & Munari, F. (1996). Monounsaturated fatty acid (avocado) rich diet for mild hypercholesterolemia. *Archives of Medical Research*, 27, 519–23.

Hoffmann, G. & Schwingshackl, L. (2012) Monounsaturated fatty acids and risk of cardiovascular disease: Synopsis of the evidence available from systemic reviews and meta-analyses. *Nutrients*, 4, 1989–2007.

## CHAPTER 6: AJI

Chan, Y. C., Chen, M. K., Lin, C. H., Lu, W. C., & Wang, C. W. (2013). Capsaicin induces cell cycle arrest and apoptosis in human KB cancer cells. *BMC Complementary and Alternative Medicine*, 13.

Derbyshire, E., Tiwari, B. K., Whiting, S. (2012). Capsaicinoids and capsinoids. A potential role for weight management? A systemic review of the evidence. *Appetite*, 59, 341–48.

Desmond, J., Kizaki, M., Koeffler, H., Kumagai, T., Lehmann, S., McBride, W., Mori, A., O'Kelly, J., & Pervan, M. (2006). Capsaicin, a component of red peppers, inhibits the growth of androgen-independent, *p53* mutant prostate cancer cells. *Cancer Research*, 66, 3222–29.

## CHAPTER 7: CAMU CAMU

Akachi, T., Kawagishi, H., Kawaguchi, T., Morita, T., Shiina, Y., & Sugiyama K. (2010). 1-methylmalate from camu-camu (*Myrciaria dubia*) suppressed D-galactosamine-induced liver injury in rats. *Bioscience, Biotechnology, and Biochemistry*, 74 (3), 573–78.

Ayala, F., Kawanishi, K., Kuroiwa, E., Moriyasu, M., Tachibana, Y., & Ueda, H. (2004). Aldose reductase inhibitors from the leaves of *Myrciaria dubia* (H. B. & K.) McVaugh. *Phytomedicine*, 11 (7-8) 652–56.

Bobbio, F. O., Cuevas, E., Mercadante, A. Z., Winterhalter, P., & Zanatta, CF. (2005). Determination of anthocyanins from camu-camu (*Myrciaria dubia*) by HPLC-PDA, HPLC-MS, and NMR. *Journal of Agricultural and Food Chemistry*, 53 (24), 9531–35.

Bradfield R, Roca, A. (1964). Camu-camu—a fruit high in ascorbic acid. *Journal of the American Dietetic Association*, 44, 28–30.

Da Silva, F., et al. (2005). Antigenotoxic effect of acute, subacute and chronic treatments with Amazonian camu-camu (*Myrciaria dubia*) juice on mice blood cells. *Food Chemistry and Toxicology*, 50 (7), 2275–81.

Dib Taxi, C. M., de Menezes, H. C., Grosso, C. R., Santos, A. B. (2003). Study of the microencapsulation of camu-camu (*Myrciaria dubia*) juice. *Journal of Microencapsulation*, 20 (4), 443–48.

Dufour, J. & Zapata, S. (1992). Camu-camu *Myrciaria dubia* (HBK) McVaugh: chemical composition of fruit. *Journal of the Science of Food and Agriculture, 61 (3)*.

Evelázio de Souza, N., Justi, K. C., Matsushita, M., & Visentainer, J. V. (2000). Nutritional composition and vitamin C stability in stored camu-camu (*Myrciaria dubia*) pulp. *Archivos Latinoamericanos de Nutrición, 50 (4)*, 405–8.

Franco, M. R. & Shibamoto, T. (2000). Volatile composition of some Brazilian fruits: umbu-caja (*Spondias citherea*), camu-camu (*Myrciaria dubia*), Araca-boi (*Eugenia stipitata*), and Cupuacu (*Theobroma grandiflorum*). *Journal of Agricultural and Food Chemistry, 48 (4)*, 1263–65.

Genovese, M., Goncalves, A., Lajolo, F. (2010). Chemical composition and antioxidant/antidiabetic potential of brazilian native fruits and commercial frozen pulps. *Journal of Agricultural & Food Chemistry, 58 (8)*.

Inoue, T., Komoda, H., Node, K., Uchida, T. (2008). Tropical fruit camu-camu (*Myrciaria dubia*) has anti-oxidative and anti-inflammatory properties. *Journal of Cardiology, 52 (2)*, 127–32.

Komoda, H., Inoue, T., Node, K., Uchida, T. (2008). Tropical fruit camu-camu (*Myrciaria dubia*) has anti-oxidative and anti-inflammatory properties. *Journal of Cardiology, 52*.

Mazza, G. (2007). Anthocyanins and heart health. *World of Food Science.* http://www.eatris.it/binary/publ/cont/369%20-%20ANN_07_54_Mazza.1201593082.pdf.

Muller, V. (2010). Camu-camu (*Myrciaria dubia*). Retrieved from http://wholeworldbotanicals .com/herbal_camucamu.

Tohi, W. (2012). The true history of camu camu, nature's most potent source of natural vitamin C. Retrieved from http://www.naturalnews.com/037389_camu_history_vitamin_C.html.

Yazawa, K., et al. (2011). Anti-inflammatory effects of seeds of the tropical fruit camu-camu (*Myrciaria dubia*). *Journal of Nutritional Science and Vitaminology (Tokyo), 57 (1)*, 104–7.

## CHAPTER 8: PURPLE CORN

Jones, K. (2005). The potential health benefits of purple corn. *Herbal Gram, 65*, 46–49.

Kang, S. W., Kang, Y. H., Kim, J. K, Kim, J. L., Lee, J. Y., Li, J., & Lim, S. S. (2012). Purple corn anthocyanins dampened high-glucose-induced mesangial fibrosis and inflammation: possible renoprotective role in diabetic nephropathy. *The Journal of Nutritional Biochemistry, 23*, 320–31.

Long, N., Naiki-ito, A., Sakatani, K., Sato, S., Shirai, T., Suzuki, S., & Takahashi, S. (2013). Purple corn color inhibition of prostate carcinogenesis by targeting cell growth pathways. *Cancer Science, 104*, 298–303.

Mazza, G. (2007) Anthocyanins and heart health. *Ann Ist Super Sanita, 43*, 369–74.

# CHAPTER 9: ARTICHOKES

Anderson, J., Baird, P., Davis, R., Ferreri, S., Knudtson, M., Koraym, A., Waters, V., & Williams, C. (2009). Health benefits of dietary fiber. *Nutrition Reviews, 67*, 188–205.

Di Venere, D., Fraioli, R., Linsalata, V., Miccadei, S., & Mileo, A. M. (2012). Artichoke polyphenols induce apoptosis and decrease the invasive potential of the human breast cancer cell line MDA-MB231. *Journal of Cellular Physiology, 227* (9), 3301–9.

Florek, E., Horoszkiewicz, M., Kulza, M., Malinowska, K., Seńczuk-Przybylowska, M., & Wachowiak, K., Woźniak, A. (2012). Artichoke—untapped potential of herbal medicine in the treatment of atherosclerosis and liver diseases. *Przeglad Lekarski, 69*, 1129–31.

# CHAPTER 10: SACHA INCHI

Beccaria, M., Cacciola, F., Dacha, M., Dugo, L., Dugo, P., Fanali, C., & Mondello, L. (2011). Chemical characterization of sacha inchi *(Plukenetia volubilis L.)* oil. *Journal of Agriculture and Food Chemistry, 59*.

Cabo, N., Chirinos, R., Gloria, P., Guillen, M. (2003). Characterization of sacha inchi *(Plukenetia volubilis L.)* oil by FTIR spectroscopy and $^1$H NMR. Comparison with linseed oil. *Journal of American Oil Chemists' Society. 80* (8).

Curb, D., Rodriguez, B., & Willcox, B. (2008). Antioxidants in cardiovascular health and disease: key lessons from epidemiologic studies. *The American Journal of Cardiology, Volume 10*.

Gomez-Pinilla, F. (2011). Collaborative effects of diet and exercise on cognitive enhancement. *Nutrition and Health, 20*.

Gutierrez, L., Jimenez, A., & Rosada, L. (2010). Chemical composition of sacha inchi *(Plukenetia volubilis L.)* seeds and characteristics of their lipid fraction. *Instituto de Ciencia y Tecnologia de Alimentos (ICTA), 30*.

Pinilla, F. (2008). Brain foods: the effects of nutrients on brain function. *Nature Reviews of Neuroscience, 9*.

# CHAPTER 11: LUCUMA

Apostolidis, E., Genovese, M. I., Lajolo, F. M., Pinto, M. da S., Ranilla, L. G., Shetty, K. (2009). Evaluation of antihyperglycemia and antihpertension potential of native Peruvian fruits using in vitro models. *Journal of Medicinal Food, 12*, 278–91.

Dini, I. (2011). Flavonoid glycosides from *Pourteria obovata* (R. Br.) fruit flour. *Food Chemistry, 124*,    884–88

Rojo, L. E., Villano, C. M., Joseph, G., Schmidt, B., Shulaev, V., Shuman, J. L., Lila, M. A., & Raskin, I. (2011). Wound-healing properties of nut oil from *Pouteria lucuma. Journal of Cosmetic Dermatology, 9* (3), 185–95.

Yao, L. H., Jiang, Y. M., Shi, J., Tomas-Barberan, F. A., Datta, N. Singanusong, R., & Chen S.S. (2004). Flavonoids in food and their health Benefits. *Plant foods for Human Nutrition, 5*, 113-22.

# CHAPTER 12: BEANS

Anderson, J., Baird, P., Davis, R., Ferreri, S., Knudtson, M., Koraym, A., Waters, V., & Williams, C. (2009). Health benefits of dietary fiber. *Nutrition Reviews*, 67, 188–205.

Arunasalam, K., Jiang, Y., Kakuda, Y., Mittal, G., Shi, J., & Yeung, D. (2004). Saponins from edible legumes: Chemistry, processing, and health benefits. *Journal of Medicinal Food*, 7 (1), 67–78.

# CHAPTER 13: PURPLE POTATOES

Furuta, S., Kobayashi, M., Masuda, M., Nishiba, Y., Oki, T., & Suda, I. (2003). Physiological functionality of purple-fleshed sweet potatoes containing anthocyanins and their utilization in foods. *Japan Agricultural Research Quarterly*, 73, 167–73.

Galli, R., Joseph, J., Shukitt-Hale, B., & Youdim, K. (2002) Fruit polyphenolics and brain aging. *Annals of New York Academy of Sciences*, 959, 128–32.

Hamouz, K. & Lachman, J. (2005). Red and purple coloured potatoes as a significant antioxidant source in human nutrition—a review. *Plant, Soil, and Environment*, 51, 477–82.

Makkieh, K. (n.d.). Purple potatoes nutrition facts. Retrieved from http://healthyeating.sfgate.com/purple-potatoes-nutrition-2182.html.

Mazza, G. (2007). Anthocyanins and heart health. *Ann Ist Super Sanita*, 43, 369–74.

Stoner, G., Wang, L. (2008). Anthocyanins and their role in cancer prevention. *Cancer Letters*, 269, 281–90.

# CHAPTER 14: CILANTRO

Aissaoui, A., Israili, Z. H., Lyoussi, B., & Zizi, S. (2011). Hypoglycemic and hypolipidemic effects of *Coriandrum sativum* L. in *Meriones shawi* rats. *Journal of Ethnopharmacology*, 137 (1), 652–61.

Anton, L., Codiță, I., Coldea, I. L., Dobre, E., Drăgulescu, E. C., Drăcea, N. O., Dragomirescu, C. C., Lixandru, B. E., & Rovinaru, C. (2010). Antimicrobial activity of plant essential oils against bacterial and fungal species involved in food poisoning and/or food decay. *Roumanian Archives of Microbiology and Immunology*, 69 (4), 224–30.

Anuradha, C. V., Deepa, B. (2011). Antioxidant potential of *Coriandrum sativum* L. seed extract. *Indian Journal of Experimental Biology*, 49 (1), 30–38.

Devkar, R. V., Desai, S. N., Gandhi, H. P., Patel, D. K., & Ramachandran, A. V. (2012). Cardio Protective effect of *Coriandrum sativum* L. on isoproterenol induced myocardial necrosis in rats. *Food and Chemical Toxicology*, 50 (9), 3150–55.

Duarte, M. C., Duarte, R. M., Figueira, G. M., Furletti, V. F., Höfling, J. F., Mardegan. R. C., Obando-Pereda, G., Rehder, V. L., Sartoratto, A., Teixeira, I. P. (2011). Action of *Coriandrum sativum* L. Essential Oil upon Oral *Candida albicans* Biofilm Formation. *Evidenced Based Complementary Alternative Medicine*, Volume 2011.

Ghorbani, A., Rakhshandeh, H., Sadeghnia, H. R. (2012). Sleep-prolonging effect of *Coriandrum sativum* hydro-alcoholic extract in mice. *Natural Product Research*, 26 (22), 2095–98.

Inbavalli, R. Sreelatha, S. (2012). Antioxidant, antihyperglycemic, and antihyperlipidemic effects of *Coriandrum sativum* leaf and stem in alloxan-induced diabetic rats. *Journal of Food Science*, 77, 119–23.

Kim, H. G., Kim, S. Y., Kim, Y. O., Oh, M. S., Park, G., & Park, S. H. (2012). *Coriandrum sativum* L. protects human keratinocytes from oxidative stress by regulating oxidative defense systems. *Skin Pharmacology and Physiology*, 25 (2), 93–99.

## CHAPTER 15: PAPAYA

Curb. D., Rodriguez, B., & Willcox, B. (2008). Antioxidants in cardiovascular health and disease: Key lessons from epidemiologic studies. *The American Journal of Cardiology*, 101.

Hernandez, C. & Hernandez, M. (2012). Papaya Power. Retrieved from: http://www.pacificnaturo pathic.com/articles/papaya_power.html.

Hewavitharana, A., Nguyen, T., Parat, M-O., & Shaw, P. (2013). Anticancer activity of carica papaya: A review. *Molecular Nutrition & Food Research*, 57, 153–64.

Ortega, M. (2012). *Effect of proteolytic enzyme and fiber of papaya fruit on human digestive health*. Retrieved from University of Illinois Dissertations and Theses.

## CHAPTER 16: YACON

Andrade, A., Guerra, N., Livera, A., Padilha, V., Rolim, P., & Salgado, S. (2011). Glycemic profile and prebiotic potential "in vitro" of bread with yacon *(Smallanthus sonchifolius)* flour. *Ciencia Y Tecnologia Alimentaria*, 31 (2).

Fernández, M., Lachman, E. C., & Orsák, M. (2003). Yacon *(smallabthus sonchifolia* (Poepp. Et Endl.) H. Robinson) chemical composition and use—a review. *Plant, Soil, and Environment*, 49, Pages 283–90.

Gorbach, S. (2000). Probiotics and gastrointestinal health. *American Journal of Gastroenterology*. 95 (1), S2–S4.

Valentová, K. & Ulrichová, J. (2003). *Smallanthus sonchifolius* and *Lepidium meyenii*—prospective Andean crops for the prevention of chronic diseases. *Biomedical Papers*, 147 (2), 119–30.

## CHAPTER 17: QUINOA

James, A., & Lilian, E. (2009). Quinoa *(Chenopodium quinoa* Willd.): composition, chemistry, nutritional, and functional properties. *Advances in Food and Nutrition Research*, 58, 1–31.

Martinez, E., Miranda, M., Puente, L., Uribe, E., Vega-Galvez, A., & Vergara, J. (2010). Nutrition facts and functional potential of quinoa *(Chenopodium quinoa* Willd.), an ancient Andean grain: a review. *Journal of the Science of Food and Agriculture, 90* (15), 2541–47.

## CHAPTER 18: SWEET POTATOES

Block, G. Vitamin C and cancer prevention: The epidemiologic evidence. (1991). *American Journal of Clinical Nutrition, 5* (1), 2705–825.

Mayne, S. Beta-carotene, carotenoids, and disease prevention in humans. (1996). *The Journal of the Federation of American Societies for Experimental Biology, 10,* 690–710.

Yanuq, S. A. C. (2008) Sweet Potato. Retrieved from http://www.yanuq.com/english/Articulos_Publicados/sweetypotatoe.htm.

# INDEX

# ⌐ ABOUT THE AUTHORS ⌐

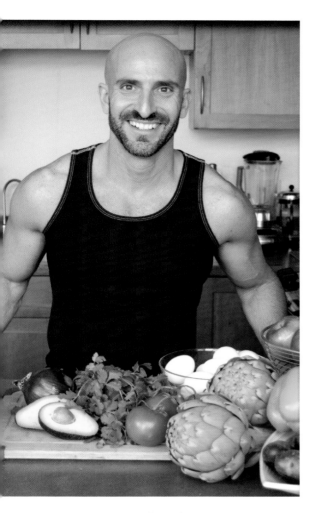

Today, **MANUEL VILLACORTA, MS, RD,** is 45 though he's far from feeling his age. He attributes his vitality to a well-balanced, healthy approach to eating, cooking, and fitness. And of course he incorporates all the power foods in this book into his diet, as well.

A nationally recognized, award-winning registered dietitian with more than sixteen years of experience as a nutritionist. Manuel Villacorta, is a respected and trusted voice in the health and wellness industry. He is the founder of Eating Free, an international weight management and wellness program, and one of the leading weight loss and nutrition experts in the country. He is the author of *Eating Free: The Carb-Friendly Way to Lose Inches, Embrace Your Hunger, and Keep the Weight Off for Good* (HCI, May 2012). Manuel served as a national media spokesperson for the Academy of Nutrition and Dietetics (2010–2013), and currently acts as a health blog contributor for The Huffington Post, an on-air contributor to the Univision television network, and a health and lifestyle contributor for Fox News Latino. Manuel is the owner of a San Francisco–based private practice, MV Nutrition, and the recipient of five "Best Bay Area Nutritionist" awards (2008, 2009, 2010, 2012, & 2013) from the *San Francisco Chronicle, ABC7,* and *Citysearch.*

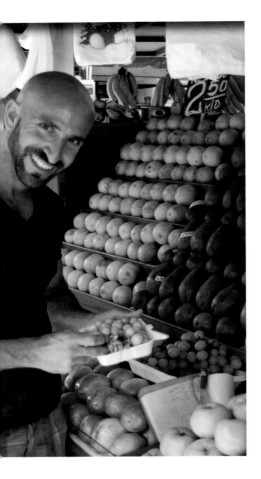

His warm, approachable style and his bilingual proficiency in English and Spanish have made him an in-demand health and nutrition expert on local and national television and radio channels, as well as in articles appearing in print publications and online.

Born and raised in Peru, Manuel makes his home in San Francisco. He earned his bachelor of science in nutrition and physiology metabolism from the University of California, Berkeley, and his master of science in nutrition and food science from San Jose State University. He has been the recipient of numerous prestigious awards for his research and contributions to the field of dietetics.

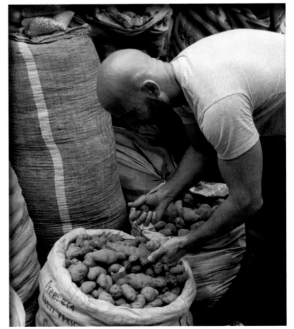

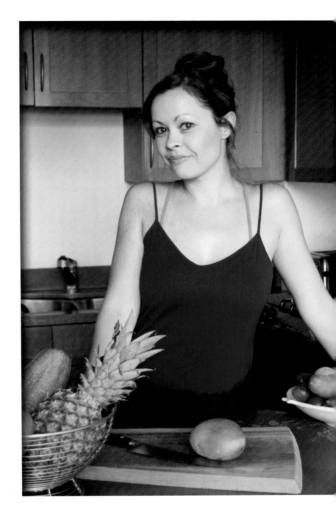

**JAMIE SHAW** is a writer, branding expert, and recipe creator, as well as a former restaurant reviewer and food blogger. An avid lover of simple, fresh ingredients and innovative preparation, Jamie specializes in projects that marry good health with great taste. In addition to supporting Manuel in his nutrition work, she consults with Urban Remedy, an international line of fruit, veggie, and nut drinks, as well as Elevated Spirits, an herbal mixology company with an Ayurvedic approach. She also serves as a ghostwriter for a variety of professional experts writing books in their respective fields.

Jamie's writing style brings personality and interest to the science of superfoods. Her knowledge of food trends added an essential ingredient in recipe co-creation for this book.

With her own business as an advertising copywriter, she's produced strategic and conceptual copy for some of the world's biggest brands, including Apple, Levi Strauss, Google, Pottery Barn, Verizon Wireless, Suzuki, Visa, and more. Over the course of her writing career, she's worked as a technical writer, a brand-namer, a copywriter, and a blogger. She also taught Creative Writing at San Francisco State University.

As an editorial writer, Jamie was a regular featured contributor for the "Two Live" Arts & Entertainment column in *The San Francisco Bay Guardian*. She also served as the North Bay dining editor for Digital City, during which time

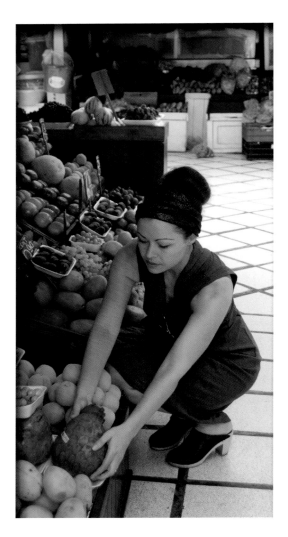

she spent a year reviewing restaurants for the 2006 "Best of the Bay" guide.

Jamie earned a BA in Creative Writing from Randolph-Macon Woman's College (now Randolph College) and an MFA in Poetry from San Francisco State University.

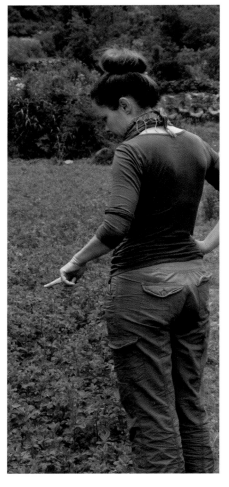